Conten

D1346924

Introduction 1

The prostate and its problems 5

Other conditions causing
'prostatic symptoms' 19

Having the prostate investigated 25

How can BPH be treated? 40

Retention of urine 56

Prostate-specific antigen 60

Prostatic cancer 67

Prostatitis and chronic pelvic pain
syndrome 102

Improving treatment 107

Questions and answers 114

Case histories 121

Useful addresses 128

Index 138

Your pages 149

About the author

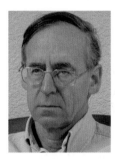

Professor David Kirk has considerable experience and interest in this field and he has recently retired from the post of Consultant Urologist at the West Glasgow Hospitals' University NHS Trust. He was also Honorary Professor at the University of Glasgow.

Introduction

Prostate problems used to be embarassing

The much repeated television series from the 1970s, *Dad's Army*, had among its platoon of characters the elderly Private Godfrey, a figure of fun who was always looking for somewhere to 'have a run out'. This contrasts with the 1990s' series *Waiting for God,* set in an old people's home, where the misery and embarrassment caused to the character Tom by his prostate problems were sympathetically dealt with, as was the enjoyment he experienced from the result of a successful prostate operation.

Situation comedies reflect real life. When Captain Mainwaring and his team, including poor old Godfrey, first entertained us, prostate disease could be a cause of embarrassed amusement, but not really something for polite conversation. It was rarely discussed openly and seriously. The symptoms produced by disorders of the prostate are embarrassing. Men brought up to be strong guys too often feel that illness, particularly one involving this part of the body, is degrading and something of which to be ashamed. Anyway, prostate symptoms are so common that most men will have friends similarly affected and may think it is just an inevitable and incurable part of growing old.

Changing attitudes

What we saw when we watched Tom's suffering was a change in the attitude of the public, the media and, it must be admitted, many doctors, to this very common problem. Now, almost every newspaper and magazine prints pieces on the prostate. Famous people who have had prostate trouble queue up to be interviewed about their experiences.

The publicity surrounding the prostatic cancer of celebrities such as David Steele and Rupert Murdoch reminds us that the prostate has a serious side. In 1997, the medical correspondent of a major daily newspaper underwent surgery for prostatic cancer, and wrote about his experiences.

Tests for prostate cancer

A test is available for the early diagnosis of prostatic cancer. In the USA there are 'Prostate Cancer Awareness Weeks' and many more men are having surgery to cure early prostatic cancer. A similar process is taking place in Britain, but more slowly.

Why is this? The media interest in 'cancer' has overshadowed the important fact – that in most men prostatic symptoms do not mean life-threatening cancer.

Symptoms are usually those of a benign condition and treatment can improve quality of life. From being neglected, prostatic disorders now have become for many an unnecessary cause of worry.

Also, as a test for cancer the PSA test is helpful but the results have to be interpreted carefully.

New treatments

A couple of decades ago, all that could be done for benign prostatic hyperplasia (BPH), the most common form of prostate disease, was an operation. This frightened many men and was one of the reasons they neglected their symptoms. Now there are new treatments and, like anything new, they have been well publicised.

This publicity has made many men, perhaps previously a bit afraid of what might happen to them, seek help. However, it also raised their expectations too much and so there has been some disappointment. For many men an operation, which need not be a fearful experience, is the best solution.

This book explains diseases of the prostate, how they cause problems and what can be done about them. Prostatic disease is not something to fear. It is not something to be ashamed of. We want fewer Private Godfreys soldiering on (in both senses) with their symptoms, fewer Toms suffering embarrassment and misery, but more Toms enjoying the pleasure of successful treatment.

KEY POINTS

■ Men with prostate symptoms should not feel embarrassed about talking over their problem with their doctor

■ Treatments are now available to improve quality of life

The prostate and its problems

What is the prostate?

What is the prostate anyway? Most people have heard of it, but have little idea what it is for, and many people don't even know where it is. Indeed doctors and scientists don't fully understand its functions, and there is still a lot to be learnt about the prostate and about the diseases affecting it.

The prostate is a gland that lies just underneath the bladder. Glands produce fluid, and the prostate gland makes part of the fluid (called semen) released at the climax of the sexual act.

The prostate needs hormones from the testicles so that it can work, and if these male hormones are low the prostate shrinks.

What does the prostate do?

The fluid from glands is made in the epithelium (layers of special cells called epithelial cells). In all glands the epithelium is surrounded by tissue called stroma. In the

The prostate and related organs

The prostate lies just underneath the bladder and surrounds the urethra. The urethra is a tube that carries urine from the bladder and also semen from the testes and prostate to the tip of the penis. The prostate produces seminal fluid which is stored in the seminal vesicles and, together with sperm from the testes, forms the semen or ejaculate.

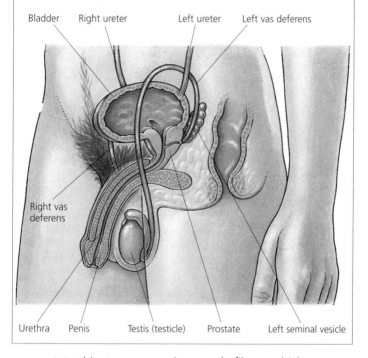

Bladder   Right ureter   Left ureter   Left vas deferens

Right vas deferens

Urethra   Penis   Testis (testicle)   Prostate   Left seminal vesicle

prostate this stroma contains muscle fibres, which can affect the symptoms produced by prostatic disorders.

Both the epithelium and the stroma increase if the prostate enlarges. In addition, although the prostate looks like a single organ, it really has two different parts which are prone to different diseases.

Although this may seem a little complicated, it is helpful to understand the problems that the prostate

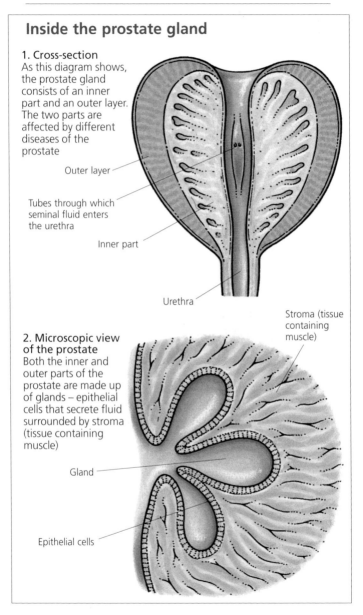

Inside the prostate gland

1. Cross-section
As this diagram shows, the prostate gland consists of an inner part and an outer layer. The two parts are affected by different diseases of the prostate

Outer layer

Tubes through which seminal fluid enters the urethra

Inner part

Urethra

2. Microscopic view of the prostate
Both the inner and outer parts of the prostate are made up of glands – epithelial cells that secrete fluid surrounded by stroma (tissue containing muscle)

Stroma (tissue containing muscle)

Gland

Epithelial cells

can cause, and how they are treated, if it is pictured as consisting of an inner and an outer part (see page 7), both of which are made up of glands (epithelium) surrounded by tissue (stroma) containing muscle.

Close to the prostate are two important muscles called sphincters. These control the bladder, stopping it leaking urine. They also help to expel the semen at the climax of the sexual act. The muscle below the prostate, called the external bladder sphincter, is particularly important for preventing leakage of urine from the bladder.

Why can the prostate cause trouble?

As a man gets older, his prostate usually becomes larger. Most of this enlargement takes place after the age of 50, so it affects mainly older men. The fact that the prostate grows is not important in itself and, indeed, the trouble it causes doesn't depend on its actual size.

However, the prostate surrounds the tube from the bladder called the urethra and as the prostate enlarges it squeezes the urethra and narrows the opening out of the bladder. This is called obstruction and it results in slowing down of the flow of urine (passing urine is sometimes referred to as 'voiding').

'Voiding' (also called obstructive) symptoms

As obstruction occurs gradually, many men do not realise that it is happening. They may notice that their urine stream does not travel as far as it did when they were younger and they may be aware that it is less forceful.

As their condition becomes worse there may be a delay in getting started (called hesitancy) and the urine

The control of urine flow from the bladder

There are two mucles called sphincters above and below the prostate. They ensure that urine is retained in the bladder until a decision is taken to void (empty) the bladder.

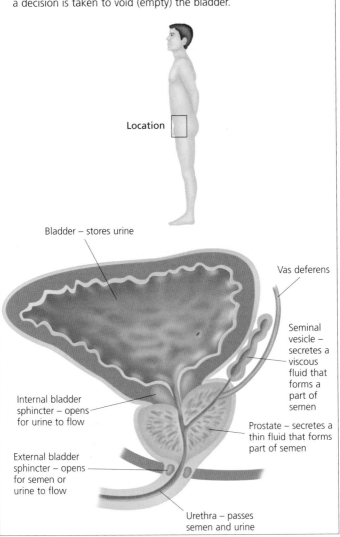

Location

Bladder – stores urine

Vas deferens

Seminal vesicle – secretes a viscous fluid that forms a part of semen

Internal bladder sphincter – opens for urine to flow

Prostate – secretes a thin fluid that forms part of semen

External bladder sphincter – opens for semen or urine to flow

Urethra – passes semen and urine

Voiding (obstructive) symptoms

When the enlargement of the prostate directly obstructs the bladder the following symptoms are likely to be experienced

Poor stream	The urine flows with less force, travelling only a short distance, sometimes straight down.
Hesitancy	Having to wait for the urine to start flowing.
Terminal dribbling	The flow of urine continues after the main stream has finished, sometimes in spurts or dribbles. Occasionally a second large volume of urine is passed (sometimes called pis en deux).
Incomplete emptying	After finishing, there is a feeling that there is still urine in the bladder.

stream tails off at the end, sometimes causing troublesome dribbling. There may be a feeling that there is still urine in the bladder – referred to as incomplete emptying.

'Storage' (also called irritative) symptoms

The obstructive symptoms described above may not be too troublesome. However, the bladder has to work harder to overcome the obstruction and, after a while, this can affect the way it behaves.

Effects of an enlarged prostate

As the prostate increases in size, so it begins to squeeze the urethra, the tube through which urine must pass in order for the bladder to empty. The effect of this is to make it difficult to pass urine and empty the bladder completely.

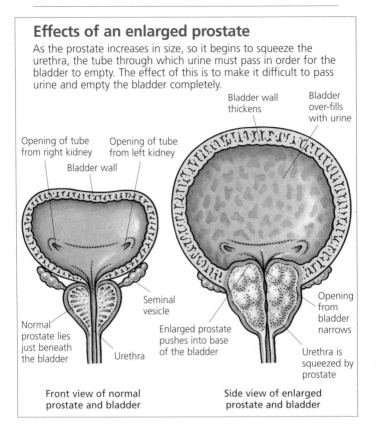

Bladder wall thickens

Bladder over-fills with urine

Opening of tube from right kidney

Opening of tube from left kidney

Bladder wall

Normal prostate lies just beneath the bladder

Seminal vesicle

Urethra

Enlarged prostate pushes into base of the bladder

Opening from bladder narrows

Urethra is squeezed by prostate

Front view of normal prostate and bladder

Side view of enlarged prostate and bladder

Some men develop storage symptoms. They need to pass urine very often (frequency) with a feeling of getting caught short (urgency) which can become so bad that wetting occurs. If these symptoms continue during the night (nocturia), loss of sleep also becomes a problem.

As Private Godfrey found, this can be a great nuisance. This is not only to the man himself, who may have to avoid long journeys and need to plan shopping trips around the local public lavatories, but also to his

Storage (irritative) symptoms

The effect on the bladder of having to work harder to overcome obstruction can produce the following symptoms.

Frequency	An abnormally short time between passing urine
Nocturia	Being woken in the night by the need to pass urine
Urgency	Being unable to hold on after feeling the need to pass urine. Can lead to urine leaking (incontinence)
Incomplete emptying sensation	With irritative symptoms, a sensation of incomplete bladder emptying sometimes occurs, even though the bladder is empty

family, friends and colleagues, who, like Captain Mainwaring, may not always be sympathetic.

In fact, friends and relatives are often more aware of the problem than the sufferer himself. He may simply slowly adjust his activities to cope with the symptoms and accept them as part of life.

Often a patient is sent to seek treatment by his wife, whose sleep is also interrupted by his repeated trips to the bathroom.

Acute retention of urine

Sometimes a man with an enlarged prostate will quite suddenly be unable to pass urine. The bladder fills up and becomes very painful. This is called acute retention and is what happened to Tom in *Waiting for God*.

Sometimes there is a reason that can be identified as the cause of retention. It is a common complication of surgical operations and even just being confined to bed, for example, by a chest infection, can be sufficient. Retention can be caused by constipation.

Some men develop retention if their bladders become overfull. This might occur, for example, on a long journey. Before motorways, hospitals on holiday routes plagued with traffic jams admitted men with retention every Saturday in the holiday season. Now that we have motorways, we still have road works and traffic jams, but the introduction of toilets on long distance coaches has made a great difference.

Cold weather is another problem. Retention occurs in men attending Easter weddings, when, perhaps after a few celebratory drinks, there will be the inevitable wait in the cold outside the church while the photographer is at work. Large drinks, especially alcoholic ones, may fill the bladder up unusually quickly. This was Tom's downfall! Drugs called diuretics, prescribed to remove excessive fluid from the body in heart or chest conditions, also sometimes cause retention.

However, retention often occurs for no apparent reason and to men who previously have not been very much bothered by their prostates – perhaps because they mainly had the less annoying obstructive symptoms. Why this should happen is not really understood. It is possible that the final stoppage results from a slight infection or something else causing swelling of the prostate.

Chronic retention

Painless retention (chronic retention) of urine occurs over months or years as the bladder slowly fills up until it may reach four or five times its normal size. Men are not usually aware that this is happening, but sometimes the overfull bladder leaks urine, causing wetness.

In a few cases, the pressure in the bladder can rise and this can damage the kidneys. This is fairly rare but, although most men with prostate disorders are very unlikely to develop kidney failure, proper treatment in the early stages will cure it completely, so it is important that tests are done to rule it out.

Other complications

If the bladder cannot empty properly, any urine left in it may become infected or might form crystals which grow into bladder stones. If the urine becomes infected, it may cause a burning sensation, called dysuria, when it is passed.

A prostate operation may be needed for repeated infections, but sometimes they are a symptom of prostatitis (see page 16).

Sometimes a large prostate can bleed, but bleeding is more likely to be the result of some other cause and must always be investigated. Very occasionally, repeated troublesome bleeding is a reason for operating on the prostate.

Why does the prostate get bigger?
Benign prostatic hyperplasia

In the majority of men, the prostate enlarges as they get older. Under a microscope this benign (simple, non-cancerous) enlargement is seen as changes called benign prostatic hyperplasia or BPH. The exact reason for this enlargement is uncertain, but it needs male hormones and does not occur in men castrated at an early age. Most men over 80 years old have the condition, and about half will have some symptoms from it.

As the prostate enlarges, both the epithelium and the stroma grow (see page 16). Sometimes the gland is not much bigger, and symptoms seem to be caused by the muscle in the stroma contracting, which constricts the bladder opening and urethra.

BPH develops in the inner part of the gland (see page 16) and, as it enlarges, it squashes the outer part of the gland into a fairly thin shell, called a capsule. BPH never spreads outside the gland.

However big the prostate, it remains covered by the capsule, rather like a chestnut in its shell. When a doctor examines a gland with BPH, it has a smooth surface with an even shape and feels rubbery, rather than hard.

Unless it causes the sort of symptoms described earlier in this chapter, the patient himself will not notice anything unusual, simply because his prostate is large, and it seems to function normally.

Cancer of the prostate

The prostate is one of the organs that can develop cancerous tumours. These usually develop in the outer part of the gland (see page 17) and may not block the urethra at first. Many men with tumours coincidently have BPH in the inner part of the gland, and often it is symptoms from this BPH that lead to the cancer being discovered.

Surrounding this outer part of the gland is a thin layer of tissue, also rather confusingly called the capsule. At first the tumour stays inside this outer capsule but, as it enlarges, it spreads through the capsule and grows into the tissue around the prostate.

Enlarged prostate caused by BPH

BPH develops in the inner part of the prostate squashing the outer part. Unless symptoms develop, such as compression of the urethra, the patient will not be aware of BPH.

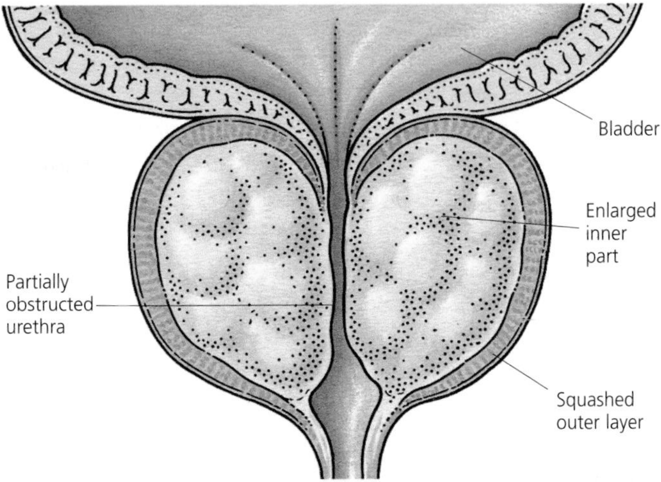

Bladder

Enlarged inner part

Partially obstructed urethra

Squashed outer layer

It may also spread elsewhere by cells breaking away from it. These are trapped by the lymph glands near the prostate and here they can grow into secondary tumours (metastases). The tumour can also spread via blood vessels, usually to the bones of the back and pelvis.

A doctor will suspect a tumour if there is a hard lump in the prostate or if the whole prostate feels hard and the shape is uneven. However, very small tumours may be impossible to feel.

Prostatitis

Inflammation of the prostate (prostatitis) from infection or other causes is not uncommon and can occur at most ages. Sometimes it causes symptoms like cystitis

Prostate cancer

Cancer of the prostate most commonly affects the outer layer of the gland, but, as a tumour grows and spreads to the central part, it will obstruct the urethra.

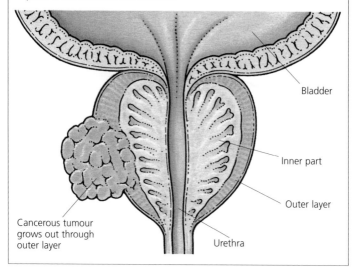

Bladder

Inner part

Outer layer

Cancerous tumour grows out through outer layer

Urethra

– such as burning pain while passing urine. In older men, it might cause a sudden increase in prostatic symptoms.

Prostatitis may cause rather vague symptoms and can be difficult to diagnose. There is more about prostatitis on page 102.

KEY POINTS

- Prostate symptoms may be 'voiding' or 'storage'

- The main disorders are benign prostatic hyperplasia (BPH), prostatic cancer and prostatitis

Other conditions causing 'prostatic symptoms'

Is it the prostate?

Although we talk about 'prostatic symptoms', trouble with urination can be caused by all sorts of things. This is one reason why GPs and hospital doctors need to do special tests to confirm that it is the prostate that is causing the trouble before advising on treatment.

Other causes of obstruction
Urethral stricture

Apart from benign prostatic hyperplasia (BPH), the condition most likely to cause blockage is a urethral stricture. This is a narrowed scarred area which can occur anywhere from just below the prostate to just inside the penis.

Strictures can result from injury – either from a direct blow, as in falling astride a fence or tree branch, or from broken bones in the pelvis that are close to the

Urethral stricture

Narrowed scarred areas of the urethra, called strictures, can restrict or obstruct the flow of urine. They can be caused by injury, such as a blow, or by infection, or by insertion of a catheter.

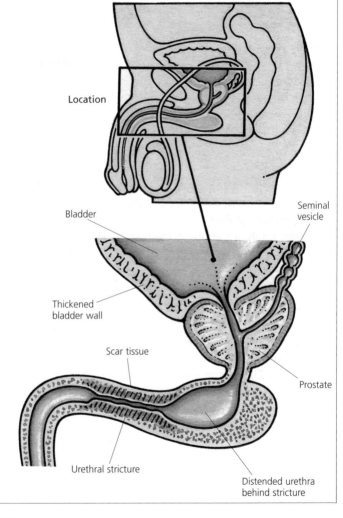

Location

Bladder

Seminal vesicle

Thickened bladder wall

Scar tissue

Prostate

Urethral stricture

Distended urethra behind stricture

bladder and urethra. They can be caused by infection, including sexually transmitted infections.

A common cause is having a small tube (catheter) put in the bladder – this is done as part of some operations, including heart surgery. A stricture can also happen after operations on the prostate itself.

What caused the stricture might have occurred many years before, so it is worth thinking about this before a hospital visit, as the doctor may ask about it. Strictures can occur at any age so they are suspected more strongly when someone has prostatic symptoms at a younger age than usual.

Stones and other bladder conditions

A stone in the bladder might cause a sudden blockage, either producing retention of urine or intermittently severe symptoms. However, a stone can itself be a complication of BPH.

Very rarely, a tumour in the bladder may grow down into the prostate, but this will usually be associated with other symptoms such as bleeding.

Causes of urinary symptoms not caused by obstruction

When symptoms are the result of prostate disease, they should not be dismissed as 'old age'. However, other conditions, not arising in the prostate, can cause similar symptoms. As people get older, all their bodily functions can deteriorate, and this includes the bladder. Storage symptoms (frequency, urgency, etc.) are most likely to occur in this way.

Effects of poor sleep

One common problem is needing to pass urine in the night. This affects elderly women as much as elderly men, and many men who have prostate operations are disappointed to find that they still have to get up in the night afterwards. Older people tend to sleep less well; they pass urine because they are awake, rather than being woken by the need to pass urine.

Effect of ageing on other organs

Sometimes the kidneys are not as good at restricting the amount of urine they make in the night, and some drugs increase the amount of urine.

Some diseases, such as diabetes, which may start in old age, can increase urine production and will affect the number of times the bladder needs to be emptied. Some diseases of the nervous system, including strokes and Parkinson's disease, can affect the bladder.

Effects of a change of lifestyle

A change in lifestyle may also cause trouble. After retiring from work, many men drink more tea or coffee than before, or visit the pub at lunchtime. More fluid in means more fluid out – hence they need to pass urine more often.

Why you should be assessed before treatment

Trouble with your bladder does not have to be an inevitable feature of getting old. However, even when it is the result of the prostate, a prostate operation is not an infallible cure for every urinary symptom, and sometimes an operation must be avoided as it might make things worse.

Before having any treatment, the condition must be properly assessed – and the next chapter explains what procedures are used to do this, why they are done and what the results mean.

Blood in the urine

It is most important that blood in the urine (haematuria) should not be considered as a 'prostate symptom'.

Up to a third of the people seen by urologists with this symptom are found to have something potentially serious – such as a tumour in the bladder or (less often) the kidney. Many of these tumours are not frankly cancerous and can be cured. In all cases, the sooner they are diagnosed, the more likely they are to be cured and the easier the treatment will be.

Blood in the urine is usually investigated either by an X-ray procedure called an intravenous urogram or by an ultrasound scan (or by both) followed by a cystoscopy (see page 36). If you see blood in your urine don't ignore it, even if it goes away – see your doctor straight away.

Sometimes, blood that is not visible to the naked eye is found when a urine specimen is tested. Although this is less likely to be the result of something serious like visible bleeding, it is still best to have it checked out.

KEY POINTS

■ Urethral strictures, stones and bladder tumours can all cause 'prostatic symptoms'

■ Deteriorating body functions associated with old age and lifestyle changes can also be called 'prostatic symptoms'

■ Blood in the urine does not usually come from the prostate and should be investigated urgently

Having the prostate investigated

Do I need my prostate checked?

If you are a man of the right age for prostate problems, having read so far you will probably be wondering whether you need to have your prostate seen to. Why not look at the questions in the box on page 26.

If you only answer 'yes' to one or two of them, you don't have much of a problem and probably don't need to worry. Your GP may arrange routine health check-ups for you, especially if you are over 75, and these may include checking the prostate. If you have bad symptoms that you have been neglecting, you certainly should do something.

How do I get my prostate checked?

You should first consult your own GP. If you seem to have a prostate problem, you will usually be referred to a urologist – a surgeon specialising not only in diseases of the prostate but also of the kidneys, bladder and male sexual organs. The urologist will need to decide:

- whether your symptoms are caused by enlargement of the prostate
- whether the enlargement is benign
- what treatment if any is needed.

Prostate self-assessment questions

If your answer is 'yes' to any of these questions then you may have a prostate problem and you should consult your doctor.

Do you think you have difficulty in starting to pass urine?	Yes	No
Do you think it takes you too long to pass urine?	Yes	No
Do you pass urine in fits and starts?	Yes	No
Do you continue to dribble urine without your full control when you have tried to stop?	Yes	No
Are you woken up from your sleep more than twice per night by the need to pass urine?	Yes	No
Do you sometimes have to rush to the toilet to pass urine?	Yes	No

This will involve you answering some questions (the history), being examined and having some special tests.

What happens if I am referred to a urologist?

Many, if not most, urology departments now have a special prostate assessment clinic. Some clinics may be run by a nurse and you will not necessarily see a doctor on your first visit.

The nurse may arrange initial investigations and probably do part of the physical examination her- or himself, and then make you an appointment to come to see the urologist on another day. It means that, when you see the urologist, the results of all your tests will be available and this usually means that a decision can be made about your treatment more rapidly.

This does, incidentally, give you an opportunity to reconsider your symptoms, because something that you may not have thought about might have been brought to your attention at this first visit. Increasingly, general practitioners, as they become more knowledgeable in looking after men with minor prostate problems, may refer you to the prostate assessment clinic and ask for the results to be sent directly back to them, so you may then not need to see a urologist.

However, you should not be concerned that this, or any delay in seeing the urologist, will cause you any harm. The clinics are carefully designed to ensure that any urgent problems are picked up and, if this should be the case, you would be given an urgent appointment. Indeed, experience suggests that men get seen more quickly in a prostate assessment clinic than by a urologist; therefore these clinics have meant that problems are picked up more rapidly than they were in the past.

The history

Knowing about a patient's symptoms is important, not only in making the correct diagnosis, but also in deciding if and how the condition should be treated. It is a good idea to think about your symptoms carefully before you see your doctor or before attending the clinic, as this will help you to answer the questions.

It is also important to make it clear why you are concerned about your symptoms. Some men simply want to be reassured that they do not have something serious, in which case, provided that all is well, they may then not want to be offered any treatment. Other men have such uncomfortable symptoms that they are desperate to have them treated.

If you are simply worried and want reassurance, do not be afraid to say this. The doctor will not mind, and it will avoid a misunderstanding which could lead to you getting the wrong advice.

Symptom questionnaires

A set of standard questions may be used either from a printed list, or sometimes from a computer. In some hospitals you may be given the questionnaire beforehand. If this happens, someone will go through the answers and deal with anything that is not clear.

The questions are designed to find out what the problem is and how severe the symptoms are. The severity is given a number and the numbers for all the questions can then be added up to give a 'score' which measures the seriousness of the problem. Questions about your general health are also important, especially if an operation is being considered.

Examination

You will need to have a general examination, including checking blood pressure. This may be done by your GP before you are referred to the hospital and you will certainly be fully examined by the urologist when you see him or her.

Your abdomen will be checked, making sure your bladder is not enlarged. Your penis and testicles will be examined. Sometimes narrowing of the opening in the foreskin – phimosis – can cause similar symptoms to those arising from the prostate, and a simple circumcision operation may be all that is needed.

The final part of the examination is feeling the prostate itself. In the past, this examination has been done only by a doctor, but now some clinics have specially trained nurses working in prostate assessment clinics to do this examination. As they are doing this all the time, they are very skilled at picking up problems in the prostate that require urgent attention.

The examination will also be done by the urologist, when you see him or her, to check the findings, and it is also often done by your GP. You have probably heard about it, and many men get worried and anxious about it. Indeed sometimes this is why men don't admit to their prostate symptoms.

It is natural to be apprehensive about this type of examination, and the person doing it knows this, realises that it is embarrassing and undignified, and will do it as discreetly as possible. If you have some problem affecting your back passage – such as piles, or pain when you open your bowels – you should mention this to the person doing the examination at the start.

Usually you will be asked to lie on your left side, although sometimes another position is preferred. It is important to relax as much as possible. Bending up your knees makes your prostate easier to feel. The person doing the examination wears a thin soft glove on which he or she puts some jelly to allow the finger to slip in easily.

The examination usually only takes a few seconds, and indicates how big your prostate is and whether it is enlarged from BPH or another cause. Normally the prostate is not tender, but if prostatitis is suspected you may be asked whether touching the prostate is painful, and very occasionally the prostate may be massaged during the examination to obtain a specimen of fluid from it. The rectum itself may also be examined.

Tests

The doctor now knows what symptoms you have, how troublesome they are, what your prostate is like on examination and how fit you are. He or she will usually have a good idea what the problem is but will want tests to confirm this and to help plan your treatment. Some tests are done in nearly all cases, others only in certain situations.

You will be asked for a sample of your urine – this might be collected when the flow test is done (see page 31). A blood sample is usually taken to check how your kidneys are working and to measure a substance called prostate-specific antigen (PSA). PSA is so important that there is a chapter about it (see page 60). The blood test results usually take a few days to come through.

Urine flow measurement

If the prostate obstructs the bladder opening, it will slow down the passage of urine. Machines that measure the flow of urine are used to test this. The test is very simple – you pass urine into a funnel-shaped container, just as if you were using a toilet, and all the measurements are done automatically.

However, the test is accurate only if a fairly large amount of urine is passed. It is a good idea to drink plenty of fluid before you go to the hospital and, if you can attend with your bladder comfortably full, so much the better.

Urine flow measurements

As a blockage of the urethra slows down the passage of urine, measurement of the flow of urine will reveal the presence of an obstruction such as benign BPH.

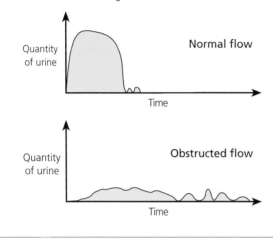

Don't worry if you haven't been able to do this – you will be given some water to drink and allowed to wait until your bladder has filled before doing the test. If, while you are in the waiting room, you feel you need to pass urine, tell one of the clinic staff. You may be able to do the flow test straight away.

Sometimes when you first do the test you might pass only a little urine. If this happens and then a few minutes later you suddenly feel the urge to go again, don't go to the toilet, but tell one of the staff so you can use the flow machine again!

When you are passing urine into the machine, relax – straining will affect the reading. Try to keep the stream in one direction; letting it 'wander' around the side may cause a false reading. You should also avoid knocking against the machine while using it. These precautions will help to produce a good record which will show if the prostate is causing obstruction or not.

One advantage of having a preliminary visit to a prostate assessment clinic is that, if any of the tests, particularly the flow measurement, have been unsatisfactory the first time, your visit to the urologist provides an opportunity for them to be repeated.

X-rays and ultrasound scans

For many patients, further tests may not be necessary, but sometimes it is a good idea to check up on the kidneys with some X-rays or scans. An X-ray called an 'intravenous urogram' or IVU, which involves an injection of a dye so that the kidneys show up on X-ray, might be done in certain circumstances. For example, it may be suggested if blood has been seen in your urine.

More often, now, if the urologist wants to look at the kidneys an ultrasound scan is used. It is very easy – a doctor or radiographer simply runs a small probe over the back and front of your abdomen.

Ultrasound can also be used to measure how well your bladder is emptying. This can be done at the same time as the kidneys are scanned. However, as there are also small portable machines designed just for this purpose, one of these might be used by either a doctor or a nurse in the clinic.

A simple X-ray of your abdomen can be useful and is particularly good at making sure that there isn't a stone in your bladder or kidneys. It also shows the size of the bladder. It is usually done after passing urine – perhaps immediately after the flow test – as another way of checking how well the bladder is emptying.

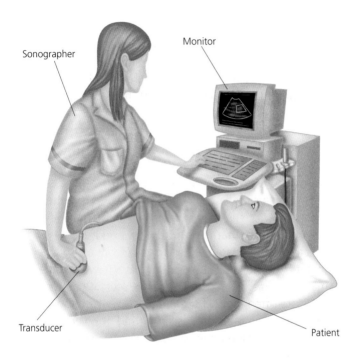

A man having his bladder scanned for residual urine

Other tests

In certain circumstances other tests might be needed.
As mentioned, an IVU may be done if there has been
bleeding or if kidney stones are suspected, or if an
abnormality is found in the kidney on an ultrasound
scan.

Transrectal ultrasound scan

A transrectal ultrasound scan (TRUS) is done using a
metal probe which is gently passed into the rectum

and allows the inside of the prostate to be examined. If necessary, a fine needle can be passed through it into the prostate to take small pieces for microscopic examination (needle biopsy).

This test will be done if an accurate measurement of the size of the prostate is needed or if cancer is suspected. Some urology clinics have a portable machine for this test and they use it on most patients with prostate disorders (see page 70).

Magnetic resonance imaging (MRI)

This way of taking images of the body is normally used when cancer of the prostate is suspected or has been diagnosed. As with a transrectal ultrasound scan, it gives a fairly accurate picture of the appearance of the prostate, but it cannot be used to take biopsies. It is also useful when spread of the cancer away from the prostate is suspected – see page 72.

To have an MRI scan, you have to lie inside a narrow metal tube for some time. It is not a good test for people who suffer from severe claustrophobia and, if this applies to you, you should mention it if such a scan is suggested. An MRI scan involves magnetism, so it is not suitable for people who have implanted devices such as heart pacemakers. When it is not possible to do an MRI scan, a form of X-ray scanning called CT (computed tomography) can be used as an alternative, although it tends to be less reliable.

Better pictures of the prostate itself can be obtained by inserting a special MRI probe into the back passage, as is done for a transrectal ultrasound scan. However, the probe used is a lot bigger and more uncomfortable. It is also quite expensive as the probe can be used only once. As there is no general agreement about the benefits of this particular form of MRI, it is still not widely used.

Cystometrogram

Fairly often an important test called a cystometrogram (or urodynamics) is needed. To do this a small tube called a catheter is passed through the urethra to measure the pressure inside the bladder. This pressure is first measured as the bladder is filled with fluid.

What does the pressure indicate?

Sometimes this test will show spasms of increased pressure, a condition called an unstable bladder, which is one cause of frequency and urgency. This is one of the things that can happen when BPH obstructs the urethra, and there is a good chance that it will improve after an operation on the prostate. On the other hand, there are other reasons for having an unstable bladder and, if it is not the result of BPH, a prostate operation will not improve it and might even make the symptoms worse.

Measuring the pressure while urine is being passed is also important. A poor flow (see figure on page 31) is usually caused by blockage from BPH. The bladder has to work harder, so the pressure in the bladder is higher than normal. However, sometimes a poor flow is not because of obstruction by the prostate, but because the bladder itself is weak – in this case the bladder pressure will be less than normal. This is another condition that will not improve after an operation on the prostate.

Sometimes the opposite might occur – the bladder will work very hard indeed, producing such a high pressure that the actual flow rate will be fairly good. Then a prostate operation is very important.

When would I have this test?

Having a cystometrogram is not very pleasant as it involves having a catheter passed into the bladder, and usually another tube is put into the back passage. You are joined up to a rather complicated looking recording machine. It is a little uncomfortable having the bladder filled up, and then passing urine with a tube still in the bladder.

For this reason it is usually advised with prostate disorders only if an operation is being considered and when results from the other simpler tests are not completely clear. It is then very important as it avoids the wrong treatment being given. As having a prostate operation is a fairly big undertaking and, as the results of the operation are not reversible, many urologists will do the operation only if a cystometrogram has first been done to show that the prostate really is causing the obstruction.

Portable device

A new method of performing a cystometrogram is being used in a few hospitals. The tubes are connected to a small portable device, attached to a belt. The patient can walk about and the measurements are done for several hours as the bladder fills and empties naturally during normal activities. This is called ambulatory urodynamics and may be used more widely in future.

Cystoscopy

Examining the bladder and prostate by looking inside it with an instrument called a cystoscope is an important test in some circumstances. It is essential if there has been blood in the urine. It may be advised if symptoms are mainly of the storage type when they might be due

Cystoscopy

A cystocope is a flexible tube which can be passed into the bladder with very little discomfort. It is used to view the internal structure of the bladder and urethra.

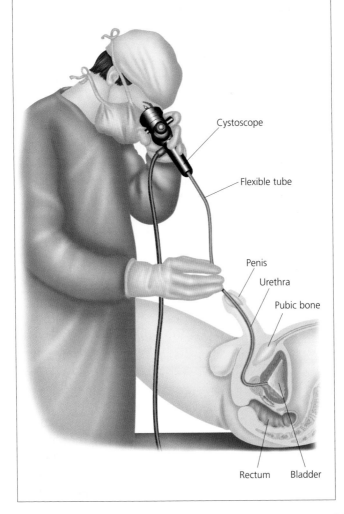

Cystoscope

Flexible tube

Penis

Urethra

Pubic bone

Rectum   Bladder

to some condition in the bladder itself. The urethra is also examined, so it is a good way of ruling out a urethral stricture.

Some surgeons find cystoscopy helpful in planning an operation, to see what the prostate looks like first. In the past, when only rigid metal cystoscopes were available, a general anaesthetic was usually given. Now, the urologist often uses a flexible cystoscope which can be passed into the bladder with very little discomfort, and a jelly containing local anaesthetic is used to numb the urethra.

The examination takes a few minutes and, because the instrument is flexible, it is even possible for the patient to see inside his own bladder! To improve the view, some fluid is run in during the examination. This may feel a little cold, but will also make the bladder feel full (which it is but not with urine!). Don't worry about having an accident – you probably won't, but if you do the examination area is designed to cope with a bit of water.

You will be asked to pass water afterwards. If you can't, or if you feel you haven't emptied your bladder properly, tell somebody – don't go home until you are comfortable.

After a cystometrogram or cystoscopy you may feel sore, have burning after passing urine, or see some blood in your urine. This settles down quickly, especially if you drink plenty for a few days. If it doesn't, or if you find it difficult to urinate, ring up the clinic or see your own GP.

KEY POINTS

■ A prostate operation is not an infallible cure for every urinary symptom. Before treatment, the condition must be thoroughly assessed

■ The doctor will want to ask you some questions, examine you and carry out some tests to assess the cause of your symptoms

■ Some of the tests, such as cystoscopy, may cause discomfort and some blood in your urine for a day or two

How can BPH be treated?

What treatments are available?

Until recently, the only real treatment for BPH was an operation. If their symptoms are not too bad, most men do not need surgery. They just need reassurance that their condition is not dangerous, and advice about simple measures such as being sensible about the amount of fluid that they drink, taking enough time to empty their bladder and learning to live with what may be only minor symptoms.

Why isn't treatment always given?

There is always a risk of side effects from any treatment (whether surgery or drugs) and, if the symptoms are mild, the side effects could be worse than the condition itself. Research has shown that operations on the prostate are usually very successful if the patient has had severe symptoms, but many men with only mild symptoms are disappointed with the result.

An operation remains the most effective method of treating BPH. An operation rather than some other type of treatment is essential if the patient has had retention of urine, or obstruction has caused kidney failure.

Sometimes the tests will show that the obstruction is so bad that an operation can prevent a complication of this type. If symptoms are very bad, an operation is usually the best way to improve them. Even if the symptoms are milder, when the tests have shown that the prostate is causing bad obstruction, an operation may be the only way of putting things right.

Compared with some types of surgery, prostate operations are really quite safe. Men with quite serious health problems can have a prostate operation without coming to harm, but an older or less fit man really should be having quite a lot of trouble to make an operation advisable.

Whether an operation is necessary often depends very much on how badly the symptoms affect the patient. Unless there is some reason why a prostate operation is essential because of a risk to health (which is unusual), you can expect the urologist to discuss it with you and he may even leave the final choice to you.

Transurethral versus 'open' surgery

The earliest operations on the prostate were done as 'open' surgery – removing the enlarged part of the gland through a surgical incision. Even today, if the gland is very large, this operation is still the best method and is usually very successful.

Just before World War II, urologists in America started doing an operation called transurethral resection of the prostate – TURP. It was one of the earliest types of minimally invasive or 'keyhole' surgery operations, and now nearly all prostate operations are done this way.

Performing a transurethral resection

A resectoscope, which is inserted through the urethra, enables the surgeon to see the enlarged prostate and then to cut away and remove the part of the gland that is causing the obstruction.

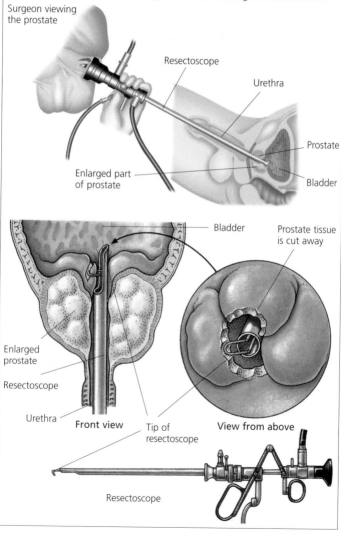

Surgeon viewing the prostate

Resectoscope

Urethra

Prostate

Enlarged part of prostate

Bladder

Bladder

Prostate tissue is cut away

Enlarged prostate

Resectoscope

Urethra

Front view

Tip of resectoscope

View from above

Resectoscope

The results of a complete resection

Resection cuts away all of the central part of the prostate gland, removing the enlarged part of the gland, increasing the width of the urethra and allowing the urine to flow more freely.

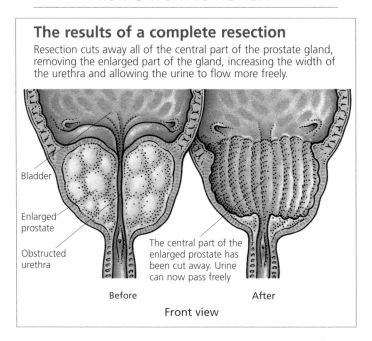

Bladder

Enlarged prostate

Obstructed urethra

The central part of the enlarged prostate has been cut away. Urine can now pass freely

Before

After

Front view

An instrument called a resectoscope is passed into the prostate along the urethra. The urologist can see the prostate through it and uses a special type of localised electric current through a metal loop to cut the prostate out in pieces. Once the enlarged prostate has been cut away, any bleeding blood vessels can be sealed, also using an electric current, leaving a cavity in the middle of the gland through which urine will pass easily.

Although the sphincter muscle around the neck of the bladder is cut away (see above), the surgeon will take great care not to injure the external bladder sphincter below the prostate, and usually control of the urine after a TURP is good. The raw cavity left at the end of the operation soon develops a protective lining called epithelium.

What happens at the time of a TURP?

The operation usually takes about half an hour. A general anaesthetic may be used, but often the operation is done with the patient awake but numb from the waist down under a spinal anaesthetic, given through a needle in the back.

Many surgeons now use a small television camera to project a picture of the operation on a screen. It is quite possible for the patient to watch his operation being done – but only if he wants to, of course.

Before you have a TURP, you will need a final physical examination, some blood tests and other tests, including a chest X-ray. The urologist and anaesthetist will discuss the operation with you. You may be given a choice between a general and a spinal anaesthetic, although sometimes, for example, with bad chest disease, a general anaesthetic might not be advisable.

To have these tests you may be admitted to hospital the day before or, alternatively, you may be seen in the outpatient department at a 'pre-admission clinic' a few days earlier. Then, it may be possible for you to be admitted to hospital on the morning of the day of your operation.

After the operation
Bleeding

At the end of the operation, a flexible tube called a catheter is put into the bladder to drain the urine; it is usually removed within two days. Although the urologist controls most of the bleeding at the end of the operation, some blood will drain with the urine, which occasionally can be quite bloody for a day or two.

Occasionally the blood will clot and block the catheter. If this happens, a doctor or nurse will clear the clot with a syringe. Many urologists use special catheters to run fluid through the bladder to reduce the risk of clotting.

Will it be painful?

You won't have any of the usual type of postoperative pain, but the catheter can be uncomfortable, and may make the bladder feel full. Sometimes painful spasms occur. If these are severe, drugs can be prescribed to control them. You will be asked to drink a lot of water each day to help flush out your bladder.

Returning to normal life

Once the catheter is removed, you should be able to pass urine almost at once. It is normal to have some frequency for a day or two, and often it is difficult to control the urine at first. A physiotherapist (or a nurse) will teach you some exercises to help control the urine.

Most men go home within a couple of days after the catheter is removed. Sometimes it is difficult to pass urine first of all, but persevering for a few hours usually does the trick. If not, the catheter sometimes needs replacing. If this happens, don't despair – usually everything is fine when it is taken out again.

Although there is no painful incision to heal up, it is important to realise that, inside, the prostate is raw and needs time to heal. This takes a few weeks, and it is important to take it easy for this time.

Continue to drink plenty of fluid (but not alcohol!). Avoid heavy lifting and don't drive for 2–3 weeks. Sexual intercourse should also be avoided for this period. You must expect to see some bits of tissue in the urine from time to time – this is like the scab coming off a skin wound and, as happens when a scab comes off, a little bleeding sometimes occurs.

Traces of blood in the urine are very common after a prostate operation. Sometimes heavier bleeding occurs, usually 1–2 weeks after the operation. Don't panic if this happens, a little blood goes a long way in the urine and often it looks worse than it is. Drink plenty and if it doesn't stop in a few hours contact your doctor.

Sometimes blood clots make it difficult to pass urine. If that happens, you might need to go back into hospital, and sometimes a catheter will be put back for a day or two. Bleeding like this almost always settles down. Sometimes it is due to an infection and antibiotics are given.

As BPH creeps up on most men unawares over some years, they are surprised by the force of their urine stream after a TURP. This usually is immediately obvious, but when frequency is the main symptom it may take longer to improve and may not return completely to normal.

Symptoms that may persist

Needing to pass urine in the night may persist after the operation because this symptom is often as much a feature of getting old as of actual prostate disease. The other symptom that may not improve is leakage at the end of passing urine. Indeed some men notice this for the first time only *after* the operation. Urine leaks out from the cavity inside the prostate. It can usually be controlled by taking a little care when passing urine.

Retrograde ejaculation

Something that almost always happens after the operation is what doctors call retrograde ejaculation. At the end of the sex act, a normal climax is felt, but nothing comes out. 'Having a dry run' describes exactly what happens. The muscle at the neck of the bladder, above the prostate, has to be removed with the prostate tissue and this means that semen leaks into the bladder rather than coming out normally. Usually, sex is otherwise unaffected, although a few men do experience difficulty in having an erection after the operation.

Settling down

After a prostate operation, your control of urine should be normal. If your symptoms before the operation were of the irritative type, leakage may occur at first and you may need some tablets to calm down your bladder, often only as a temporary measure. More rarely the lower sphincter muscle is weakened by the operation. This will usually improve with muscle-strengthening exercises. It is very unusual for this to be permanent, but operations can be done to put it right if all else fails. Leakage can occasionally result from insufficient prostate being cut away and the bladder not emptying completely. If so, a second TURP might be needed.

Men who have had a TURP are among the most satisfied customers seen in a urology clinic. The majority are delighted with the operation. A few are disappointed with the result – often those whose symptoms were fairly mild before the operation and who find that side effects, such as those above, are worse than their original symptoms.

A poor result from a TURP usually means that the operation was not the best treatment for that patient, rather than anything having gone wrong with the operation itself. That is why it is important for the right tests to be done beforehand and why the patient often must decide for himself if his symptoms are worth the discomfort of an operation and the risk of side effects. Above all, it is important to go to a urologist expecting to be given helpful advice but not necessarily to have an operation.

Drug treatment of BPH

For men with prostate symptoms who are not badly affected, who do not want to consider surgery and who are not fit enough for an operation, there is an alternative. BPH can now be treated with drugs.

There are two sorts of drug – one makes the prostate smaller and the other relaxes the muscle in the prostate and bladder neck. Both types of drug can reduce the obstruction caused by the prostate sufficiently to relieve the symptoms.

Hormone treatment

The drugs that shrink the prostate interfere with the action of the male hormone, testosterone, which is part of the cause of BPH. This reverses the condition and the prostate shrinks. Male hormones work in a different way in other organs, so this type of drug affects only the prostate and is almost completely free of side effects.

A number of these drugs are being developed, and two are now in use:

- finasteride (Proscar)
- dutasteride (Avodart).

Both are given as a single tablet once a day.

It is important to realise that it may take three months or more before the prostate shrinks enough to improve the symptoms, so this type of drug is prescribed as a long-term treatment. Don't stop taking it after a week or two because it doesn't seem to be working.

Although it is very safe and free from side effects, a small number of men do experience failure of erections or other sexual difficulties. This usually improves if the drug is stopped. If sex is very important, you might feel that this treatment is not right for you – although sexual problems are *more* common after a TURP and then are not reversible.

The other important point about this type of drug is that, as soon as it is stopped, the prostate grows back to its original size very rapidly – so once it has worked, keep on taking it.

As this type of drug causes the prostate to shrink, it also reduces the amount of blood that is flowing through it. This can be effective in preventing bleeding from the prostate which can occasionally be a troublesome symptom, especially in men who have had TURP operations and in whom the prostate has regrown a little afterwards. Thus, although the main indication for this type of drug is still to treat prostatic symptoms, it is also used to treat bleeding from the prostate, but only after other causes of bleeding have been ruled out.

Finasteride and dutasteride can reduce PSA levels in the blood (see page 60). If you have been taking either of these drugs your doctor will take this into account when assessing your PSA test results.

Alpha-blocker drugs

The other type of drug used for treating BPH is called an alpha blocker. The prostate contains muscle, contraction of which narrows the opening of the bladder and increases any obstruction caused by BPH. Alpha blockers relax the muscle, reduce the obstruction and so improve the symptoms.

Unfortunately these drugs also affect muscle in other parts of the body, especially in blood vessels, and can cause side effects such as faintness, weakness and lethargy. This type of drug is also used to treat high blood pressure, but some of the newer ones seem to act more on the prostate than other organs and may have fewer side effects.

Their big advantage is that they work almost immediately. At present, prazosin (Hypovase), indoramin (Doralese), terazosin (Hytrin), alfuzosin (Xatral), doxazosin (Cardura) and tamsulosin tablets (Flomaxtra XL) and tamsulosin capsules (various brands) are in use. They differ in how often they need to be taken and some of them need to be built up from a small dose. Their side effects differ – so if one isn't suitable, it is worth trying another.

Alpha blockers can cause retrograde ejaculation, but this will revert to normal if the drug is stopped. Just as with hormone treatment, the rate of urinary flow is only slightly improved.

Choice of drug

Choosing which of these two types of drug to use depends on a number of things.

Some men, often those whose symptoms occur at a youngish age, don't have much actual enlargement of the prostate. For them, the action of the prostatic muscle seems to be the main cause of the obstruction, and so an alpha blocker is the best choice.

If a man with a prostate like this does need an operation, the surgeon may not have to cut away any prostate, but may just make an incision in one or two places to open it up. The patient himself won't really be able to tell much difference from an ordinary TURP.

Hormone treatment with finasteride or dutasteride probably should be prescribed only when the prostate is definitely enlarged. It seems that, the bigger the prostate, the more effective these drugs will be. As it takes some time to shrink the prostate, the patient must be prepared for this.

Combined treatment

Recently, reports of a study looking at the use of these two different types of drug given together have suggested that the combination of both types of drug, at least in some circumstances, might be more effective. Sometimes, because they work faster, an alpha blocker is given in addition to finasteride or dutasteride for a few months at the start of treatment.

When is drug treatment used?

Drug treatment is usually suggested if symptoms are mild, the obstruction is not too bad and there is no reason to avoid a particular drug. Drugs may be tried in more severe cases if there are medical reasons to avoid surgery. If an operation has to be delayed, either because of a long waiting list or because it is not convenient at the time, drugs can be used for temporary help.

Some men close to retirement might want to wait until they stop work to have an operation. University or school teachers, politicians or other men with fixed vacations might prefer an operation during the summer and find temporary drug treatment helpful.

Occasionally the urologist might suggest trying some drug treatment first to see if it helps a particular symptom before taking the irreversible step of an operation.

Although these drugs can relieve symptoms in men for whom an operation isn't appropriate, there are still many men who are best advised that they do not really need any treatment. Also, drugs should ideally be used only after the prostate has been properly assessed and the tests described earlier have been done. Often this still means seeing a urologist but, partly as a result of the introduction of drugs to treat BPH, many GPs are becoming more involved in treating the prostate.

Other treatments

A lot of publicity has been given to heat and laser treatment for BPH, so much so that patients are often disappointed when they find that they cannot have this done in their local hospital.

Heat

Heat treatment (hyperthermia or thermotherapy) heats up the prostate. The treatment is given through a probe placed either in the back passage or in the urethra.

Early types only warmed up the prostate a little bit and had a pretty small effect, although patients' symptoms often improved. It is now possible to heat up the prostate a lot more without affecting the surrounding organs, and the results are more promising. The effects are probably closer to those produced by drugs than by a TURP, and heat treatment is unlikely to become an alternative to TURP for men with severe BPH.

Laser

Laser treatment is more like a TURP, and is an alternative way of removing the enlarged part of the prostate, or of simply cutting it open to widen it. There are a number of different ways of applying laser treatment. Although laser treatment in medicine is topical and receives much publicity, urologists have yet to agree on the best way to use lasers on the prostate, or even whether it will prove to be a useful treatment in the long run.

A technique called 'green light laser treatment' has been developed in the USA. A drug sensitises the prostate tissue so that the laser light will selectively destroy it. Although this is attractive, more investigation is needed before it can be used as a routine treatment.

There is now a similar treatment called vaporisation, which uses a slight modification of the resectoscope instrument used for a TURP. Of these newer methods of treatment, some type of laser technique is most promising, but it will be some time before the tried and tested TURP is replaced.

The advantage of many of these treatments is that they can be performed as day-case surgery. However, it is often necessary for the patient to have a catheter in the bladder for several days after treatment and the long-term effects are uncertain. Just because they are 'new', they are not necessarily better.

Although their advantages and disadvantages are becoming understood, most urologists still feel that these new treatments need more testing before they can be generally recommended.

Why are new treatments not available everywhere?

The equipment needed for many of these new treatments is expensive. This prevents it being available in every hospital, and means that, although the treatment may be offered to patients in some areas, it will not be available in others.

This does have an advantage – a number of urologists with a special interest in this type of treatment are carefully evaluating it. When we know how well the treatment works, that will be the time when each area of the country can decide whether it is worth spending the money necessary to make the treatment generally available. Where such a treatment is suggested, it may be as part of the trial comparing it with another treatment. There is more about trials for prostate disease on page 109.

Stents

Stents are short tubes, usually made of inert metal mesh, which are placed in the prostate to keep it open. They can be put in with very little disturbance, often under local anaesthetic. A stent might be used in a man who is too unfit for an operation, to avoid him having to have a permanent catheter. However, they can often cause long-term problems and are used less now than a few years ago.

Herbal or 'natural' remedies

There are a lot of preparations said to help prostate disease, which can be purchased directly from a chemist or health food store; some are advertised in newspapers and magazines. They may include substances that do help, but will not have been tested as thoroughly as the drugs described in this chapter.

Different preparations of the 'same' substance could differ in strength and content. These 'drugs' might help, and probably do no harm. However, if you do decide to use one of them, it is important that you tell your GP or urologist. They are not a substitute for conventional treatment, especially for cancer, and it is important that you don't stop any treatment prescribed by your GP or specialist.

KEY POINTS

- Surgery is the most effective way to treat BPH and transurethral resection of the prostate (TURP) is now the operation of choice

- The benefits of surgery have to be weighed against the side effects and possible complications

- Drug therapy is available for men whose symptoms are mild, who do not want to consider surgery or who are not fit enough for an operation

- The two main types of drug are those that shrink the prostate (hormone treatment) and those that relax the muscle within the prostate (alpha blockers)

Retention of urine

Acute retention of urine

Acute (sudden-onset) retention of urine is one of the most unpleasant things that can happen to a man with prostate trouble. He feels the need to pass urine but when he gets to the toilet he can force out only a dribble or nothing at all.

As his bladder fills, it becomes more and more painful. Occasionally, after a long period of discomfort, something finally comes out and the condition rights itself.

Often it doesn't, and this means a trip to hospital to have a catheter put into the bladder to drain the urine. This sounds a bit unpleasant but it is so effective that many doctors consider it to be the most worthwhile thing they can do for a patient.

Catheterisation

Putting a catheter in is called catheterisation. Before the catheter is inserted, some jelly containing a local anaesthetic is put into the urethra. This numbs it and makes it slippery to help the catheter go in.

After a short delay to let the anaesthetic work, the doctor passes the catheter in a sterile manner. There is usually a dodgy moment as the catheter goes through the prostate into the bladder, but then the relief is instant.

Sometimes the catheter won't pass. If this happens, a suprapubic catheter is used. This is put into the bladder through the skin of the lower abdomen under local anaesthetic. Although this sounds awful, the full bladder is so close to the skin that it really is very safe and straightforward.

Usually the patient is then kept in hospital, although it is quite possible to go home with the catheter. If the patient lives in a remote place, his GP might catheterise him at home to avoid a long and painful ambulance journey.

The catheter might be taken out after a few days, particularly if there is an obvious cause for retention (such as constipation or an alcoholic binge) and quite a few men can then pass urine again. One of the alpha-blocker drugs (see page 49) is sometimes prescribed to help the patient to pass urine when the catheter is removed.

However, retention often means that a prostate operation is on the horizon, and frequently it will be done as soon as there is a space available in the operating theatre.

Chronic retention causing renal failure

Sometimes, painless chronic (long-term) retention is associated with kidney failure. In this case the treatment is a little different. A catheter is still necessary, but once the blockage is removed the kidneys start to produce copious amounts of fluid and this must be replaced.

How a catheter works

Catheterisation involves passing a tube up the penis into the
bladder and inflating a small balloon to keep it in place. It sounds
unpleasant, but it provides an immediate solution to an
uncomfortable condition.

Location

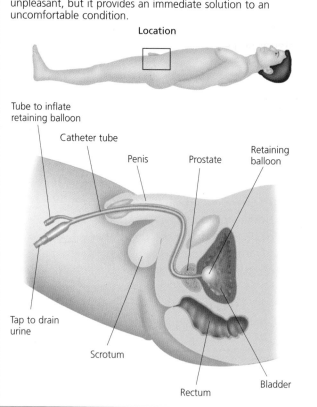

Tube to inflate
retaining balloon

Catheter tube

Penis

Prostate

Retaining
balloon

Tap to drain
urine

Scrotum

Rectum

Bladder

This usually means having a drip into a vein in the
arm. Before going on to have a prostate operation, the
kidneys have to recover and this could take a few weeks.

Results of treatment

After sudden acute retention, the results of prostate
surgery are usually very good. When chronic retention

is long term, the overstretched bladder may not work very well and, even after a good operation, will still not empty. Sometimes the bladder improves if a catheter is left in for a few weeks – this does not mean having to stay in hospital, as it is quite easy to look after a catheter at home.

KEY POINTS

- Retention of urine can be relieved by insertion of a catheter into the bladder to drain the urine

- After catheterisation for retention, a prostate operation is often required

Prostate-specific antigen

Why is prostate-specific antigen significant?

In the 1990s, a blood test called prostate-specific antigen (PSA) test was introduced. This has been given a lot of publicity as a method of diagnosing prostate cancer at an early stage when it can be cured. There is more to it than that, and understanding this test and its significance is important.

PSA is a substance made only by the prostate gland and is part of the fluid that the prostate adds to the semen. Some PSA gets into the blood and the amount in the blood can be measured. All men have PSA in their blood.

So, having PSA in your blood is normal for a man. When a doctor does a PSA test, he wants to know how much PSA there is. Think of the PSA in the blood as if it is 'leaking' out of the prostate. More PSA will come from a large prostate than from a small one, so as you get older your PSA can increase as your prostate enlarges.

When is PSA high?

Some diseases of the prostate make it more 'leaky' and, in this case, the amount of PSA is even higher. This happens with cancer of the prostate and is the reason why the test can be used to look for cancer. Other diseases of the prostate also make it more leaky – for example, the PSA may be high when the prostate is infected. It also goes up after a prostate operation, or even simply following a cystoscopy examination or having a catheter passed.

As older men have larger prostates and also more have non-cancerous diseases of the prostate such as prostatitis, the average PSA is higher in men of 75 than in men of 55. So if your PSA is higher than 'normal' it doesn't mean you have cancer. You might have, but it is more likely that you have BPH, or that something else has happened to push up the amount of PSA in your blood.

PSA and diagnosis

As a test for cancer, PSA is helpful but the results have to be interpreted carefully. In technical terms it is not very specific and it gives a lot of false positives – results that seem to indicate cancer but which on further investigation do not. If PSA is very high, this does usually mean there is cancer. If it's only a little bit raised, the size of the prostate and any other conditions affecting the prostate must be taken into account. It will certainly be necessary to do more tests before cancer can be diagnosed.

The diagnosis is usually confirmed by taking some small pieces of prostate (a biopsy) with a needle, usually when a transrectal ultrasound scan (TRUS) is done (see page 33). Sometimes this can cause infection in the urine or even the bloodstream. More importantly, the biopsy might miss the tumour, so that a negative biopsy gives a false picture. This means that, even if the biopsy is negative, it is usually necessary to have further PSA checks and even another biopsy. It can be very difficult to be completely certain that a raised PSA is not caused by cancer.

One new development may reduce some of this uncertainty. It is now realised that there are at least two types of PSA in the blood and one of these types is increased when the PSA is raised as a result of BPH.

Measurement of the proportion (ratio) of these different types of PSA gives some guidance as to whether an increase in PSA is likely to result from BPH or cancer. This can be quite helpful (for example, if someone has had a biopsy that is negative), but the difference is still not entirely clear cut. A test that accurately indicates cancer has still to be discovered, but research is progressing in this area.

PSA and cancer

In a man who is found to have cancer of the prostate, the amount of PSA is a good guide to the extent of his disease, and helps in deciding how he should be treated. If the PSA is normal (and one problem is that a man with cancer of the prostate can have a normal PSA) or only slightly raised, it is unlikely that the tumour has spread significantly and this is reassuring.

At the other extreme, a very high level of PSA is sufficient to make a diagnosis of cancer of the prostate. In these circumstances, it is often possible to save the patient the discomfort and the delay of having further tests done by arranging for his treatment to be commenced as soon as possible. Successful treatment of cancer of the prostate will lower the PSA, and regular checks on the amount of PSA in the blood are an important part of the follow-up.

Screening for cancer of the prostate

Cervical smears are used to screen for cancer of the cervix in women. Can PSA be used as a test to screen for cancer of the prostate in the same way?

This is a difficult question to answer because there may be no clear difference in the levels of PSA found in the blood of men with cancer and the amount in the blood of men with simple BPH and other benign conditions. In America it is now very popular for men to have their PSA checked once a year.

Why don't we screen men in Britain?

It is natural for men in Britain to wonder why screening is not done here as a routine procedure – they may have a cancer causing no symptoms, which could be cured if it was diagnosed early.

The issue is complicated and there is still a debate whether a national screening programme for men using the PSA test would ultimately cut deaths from prostate cancer.

In the first place, for everyone who has cancer diagnosed in this way, many others will have to have tests done, and will experience a lot of worry waiting for the results. If cancer is found, a radical prostatectomy (or perhaps radiotherapy) will be necessary to get rid of the cancer, and this is a fairly serious operation.

All this would be worthwhile if it produced a large reduction in the number of men dying from cancer of the prostate. However, some very early cancers grow slowly and in many cases might never cause harm, so it isn't too clear how many lives would be saved. This is especially the case with older men – so, although it might be a good idea to check the PSA in a man aged over 55, it is less likely to be done in men aged over 75.

In fact, by the age of 80, over half of all men will have some cancer cells in their prostate, but few will die as a result of the cancer.

As a number of men with cancer can have quite a low PSA, there has been a trend, particularly in the USA, to lower the level of PSA above which a biopsy is advised. It is certainly true that this helps to diagnose more cancers. However, a well-known American urologist, Dr Thomas Stamey, who had done a lot of the early research work on PSA, has written about his concerns. He thinks that many of these extra cancers being diagnosed may not be potentially harmful and are being treated unnecessarily.

Research into better tests

It is for these reasons that most specialists think it is too early to recommend screening of men without prostate symptoms, but research into the value of screening is going on. PSA is not an ideal test, and newer ones are being developed, one of which is done on urine rather than blood. A test that identified cancer more accurately would certainly help, but perhaps more important is to be able to identify those tumours that are dangerous and need treatment, and avoid unnecessary treatment of men whose cancer is unlikely to harm them. It would then be easier to recommend screening. It would also be easier if there were a simpler treatment than radical prostatectomy (see page 72).

PSA test on request

Many patients are interested in having their PSA measured because they are concerned about the possibility of having prostate cancer.

However, it is recommended that, before a man has his PSA tested, he be fully informed of the various issues raised in this chapter, and it will probably become standard practice for men to be given information leaflets to read before they finally decide to have a PSA test performed. If you have thought of having your PSA measured to check up whether or not you might have prostate cancer, the information you have already read in this chapter might give you some help in deciding.

Provided that you are aware that there are disadvantages as well as advantages (and there are some men who have had the test done who now regret having done so), you should discuss it with your doctor. He or she may want to give you further information, before having the test.

As a general rule, it is probably wise to measure the PSA in a man who has prostatic symptoms, as such symptoms can be the result of cancer of the prostate and, if they are, they may need different treatment than if they were caused by BPH. Because of this, most British urologists are seeing more men with prostatic cancer.

The chapter on cancer describes the operation of radical prostatectomy for early cancer. Fifteen years ago this operation was not often done in the UK and would have received only a brief mention. It is now part of the regular treatment in many urology departments, largely because of earlier diagnosis through using the PSA test.

KEY POINTS

■ The prostate-specific antigen (PSA) test is a test for assessing prostate disease

■ Many factors, other than cancer, can increase the level of PSA in the blood

■ Use of the PSA test is leading to more men with prostatic cancer being treated

Prostatic cancer

A common but treatable cancer

Cancer is an alarming word. Many men fear that their prostatic symptoms are caused by cancer. In most cases, this fear is unfounded, but it is true that cancer of the prostate is quite common and, like most types of cancer, it can be fatal. However, it is a form of cancer for which many types of treatment are available. Also, it often grows slowly and may cause little harm, especially in very elderly men.

Recently, doctors have discovered new ways of detecting early cancers in the prostate. This means that more men with prostatic cancer are being diagnosed at an earlier stage.

As mentioned in the last chapter, there is much debate amongst specialists about whether these tests should be used for screening in the way that women are screened for breast and cervical cancer (see page 63).

Is it inherited?

Why cancer of the prostate is so common is not

known. In most cases there is no clear family history, but there is a form of the disease which does seem to run in families. If you have had a single relative with the disease, don't worry. However, if two closely related relatives have had cancer of the prostate, particularly if it was when they were fairly young, it is worth getting your prostate checked from time to time after you reach 50.

What triggers it?

There are differences between races and in different parts of the world, some of which might be the result of diet or environmental factors. For example, prostatic cancer is uncommon in Japan, but Japanese men who live in America have a higher risk of developing it. This is probably as a result of differences in diet. Certain types of fatty food may predispose to prostate cancer, whereas other foods, possibly including soya products, are protective. It is still too early to give definite advice but, as we understand more about these differences, it may become possible to advise on diets that reduce the risk of prostatic cancer.

Although there was some recent concern that having a vasectomy might make cancer of the prostate more likely, most experts are now agreed that this is not so.

The difference between cancer of the prostate and benign enlargement (BPH) is that the cancer can grow out from the prostate into the surrounding tissues. It can also spread to other parts of the body (metastases), particularly to the bones where it can cause pain or even fractures.

When cancer is the cause of prostatic symptoms, these can come back after treatment if the cancer grows again. Sometimes, cancer in the prostate itself may not cause any symptoms, and the first sign of the disease might arise in some other part of the body.

Diagnosis of cancer

Your doctor may suspect that there is a tumour in your prostate if it feels abnormally hard or irregular, or if your prostate-specific antigen (PSA) level (see page 60) is particularly high. When either of these is found, the doctor will often arrange for you to have a transrectal ultrasound scan (TRUS), so that some biopsies (pieces of tissue) can be taken for pathological examination.

Diagnosing from tissue samples

Sometimes the patient will need a transurethral resection of the prostate (TURP, see page 41) anyway, because of the severity of his prostate symptoms. As TURP removes tissue that can be examined, it will be done promptly if cancer is suspected – as a way of clarifying the diagnosis. Sometimes cancer is not suspected – and it is diagnosed only when the tissue that is removed at an operation is examined by a pathologist.

How fast will it grow?

In addition to diagnosing whether there is cancer in the prostate, the appearance of the tumour can give some guidance as to how rapidly it is likely to grow. The pathologist will usually give what is called the 'Gleason score'. This is a number from 2 to 10. The higher the score, the more likely the cancer is to grow rapidly and to spread. If a patient has a tumour with a high score he will usually be advised that early treatment is important.

Transrectal ultrasound scan (TRUS)

An ultrasound probe is inserted into the rectum. An image of the internal structures is produced from the sound waves. A fine needle may be guided to the prostate to remove tissue samples.

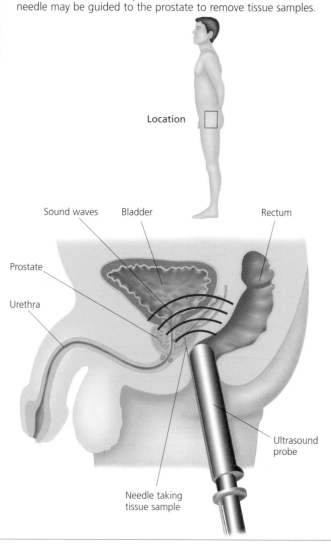

Location

Sound waves

Bladder

Rectum

Prostate

Urethra

Ultrasound probe

Needle taking tissue sample

Checking the tumour has not spread

An X-ray, or (more usually) a test called a bone scan, is done to check that there has been no spread to the bones. This is done by injecting a small amount of a radioactive substance. It is taken up where the bone is active and is detected by a special scanner.

This is not a specific test for cancer and uptake might be the result of other conditions such as arthritis, old healed fractures and benign diseases of the bones. X-rays of the abnormal areas may help. The best test is probably magnetic resonance imaging (MRI). However, this will be recommended only in certain cases, especially if there is a worry that cancer in the spine is pressing on nervous tissue. Very occasionally an orthopaedic surgeon might be asked to take a small piece of bone from the area that is abnormal on the scan. This will be examined under a microscope to see what is causing the abnormality. MRI is also used to give a more accurate picture of the prostate itself before radical prostatectomy or radiotherapy.

How is cancer of the prostate treated?

Removing or destroying a cancerous growth will cure the disease, provided that it has not spread. Until recently this was all that could be done for most cancers and, if spread (metastases) had already occurred, little more could be done.

However, there are now many treatments available that can be used to destroy or shrink cancer that has spread to other parts of the body. As we will see, cancer of the prostate was one of the first types of cancer for which treatment of this type was developed.

Magnetic resonance imaging (MRI)

Magnetic resonance imaging (MRI) uses powerful magnets to align the atoms in the part of the body being studied. Radiowave pulses break the alignment causing signals to be emitted from the atoms. These signals can be measured and a detailed image built up of the tissues and organs.

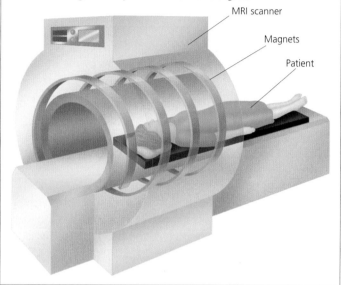

MRI scanner

Magnets

Patient

Removal of the prostate – radical prostatectomy

Most people expect cancer to be treated by surgical removal of all or part of the organ in which it occurs, as in cancer of the breast in women, cancer of the testis, cancer of the kidney and many other types of the disease. A famous urologist called Hugh Hampton Young working at the Johns Hopkins Hospital in America first described radical prostatectomy in 1905. The operation removes the whole prostate gland and is becoming more common in the UK for men with cancer of the prostate.

What happens in a radical prostatectomy?

This operation consists of removing the whole of the prostate gland and the seminal vesicles, and then reconnecting the urethra to the bladder. This procedure is usually performed only on younger patients.

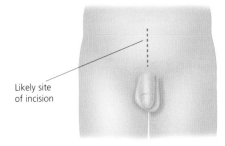

Likely site
of incision

Point of incision for surgery

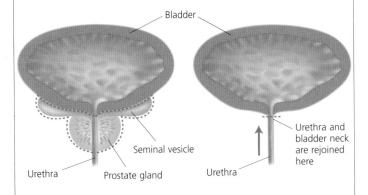

Bladder

Seminal vesicle

Urethra   Prostate gland

Urethra and
bladder neck
are rejoined
here

Urethra

**Parts that are removed in
a radical prostatectomy**

**Situation after the completion
of a radical prostatectomy**

The reason that it is not done in more cases is that cancer of the prostate can be difficult to detect until it has grown outside the prostate gland. Once this has happened, it is impossible to remove all the cancer by surgery and so an operation will not cure the disease.

Also doctors can now diagnose cancers at an earlier stage. Many small early cancers grow very slowly and can take as long as ten years to cause trouble. Obviously, for a man aged, say, 85 years, this sort of tumour is not going to be dangerous and at this age he would not stand up to major surgery very well.

For this reason, removing the prostate as a treatment for cancer is usually only done in younger patients and when there is reason to believe that the cancer is going to grow fairly quickly. Usually the operation is recommended only for men who have a life expectancy of more than 10 years.

Laparoscopic radical prostatectomy

As with many surgical operations previously done through an open incision, some surgeons are now removing the prostate using a laparoscope (keyhole surgery). Besides the usual benefits of this type of surgery – less pain, shorter time in hospital and quicker recovery – laparoscopic radical prostatectomy has other advantages.

As the surgeon can see into the pelvis more clearly, certain parts of the operation can be done differently. In particular, the urethra can be stitched on to the bladder more thoroughly, so that there is less chance of urine leaking, and the catheter can be removed sooner.

On the other hand, most men find that they get over an open radical prostatectomy quite quickly and the advantages of laparoscopy may be less than with some other operations. Also, some surgeons are concerned that the laparoscopic operation might not be quite as thorough in clearing the cancer.

Laparoscopic radical prostatectomy is very skilful, requiring a lot of training and experience and it is certainly going to be a long time before there are enough trained surgeons for this approach to be widely available. By then the operation will have been done for long enough to be sure that it is as effective as the open operation.

A method has now been developed, called robotic prostatectomy, in which the surgeon operates, by remote control, the laparoscopic instruments actually being held in a complicated machine. This is now being done in a few centres in the UK. The equipment is very expensive, and the technique has to be learnt by the surgeon. Although it has had a lot of publicity in the press, it is unrealistic to expect this operation to become widely available; nor should it be available until experience shows that the results are as good as with 'normal' surgery.

Radiotherapy – external beam treatment

This treatment can destroy small tumours and thus cure the cancer, so it is an alternative to radical prostatectomy. It may be suggested if the patient is not fit for an operation, and some men choose it in preference to surgery. Although removing a tumour completely by an operation may seem more satisfactory, there is no definite proof that one treatment cures the disease better than the other.

Radiotherapy can also be used when surgery is not possible because the cancer has spread outside the prostate. Here it may not 'cure' the cancer but, by shrinking it, it will prevent it from causing trouble and may reduce the chances of it spreading further.

Radiotherapy – external beam treatment

Three dimensional radiation therapy allows doctors to increase the doses of radiation delivered to the prostate gland without increasing damage to nearby tissues. Before treatment is begun digital images of the prostate are prepared that are synchronised with the delivery of radiation beams.

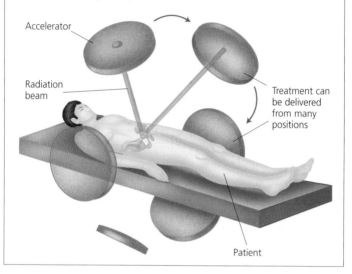

Accelerator

Radiation beam

Treatment can be delivered from many positions

Patient

New methods of giving radiotherapy – conformal radiotherapy and intensity-modulated radiotherapy (IMRT) – have been developed that concentrate the radiation on to the tumour. This makes it more effective at destroying the cancer, and also reduces the risk of radiation damaging the surrounding normal organs.

Radiotherapy – brachytherapy

The main problem with radiotherapy is that it not only affects the tumour but also reaches the surrounding organs – in the case of the prostate the rectum (back passage) and the bladder. In the short term this will affect them, causing temporary bowel and bladder

Radiotherapy given out by 'seeds' in brachytherapy

The graph shows how the radioactivity from the seeds implanted in the prostate is delivered to the diseased tissue slowly over a period of months. A large amount is delivered at first; by six months about 85 per cent has been given and it has almost all gone at the end of a year.

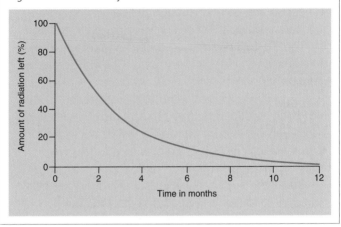

upsets. Occasionally it produces permanent damage, with more serious consequences. These risks can be reduced by the new technique of 'conformal radiotherapy' (see page 82) and/or by shrinking the tumour with preliminary hormone treatment (see page 88).

However, there is a different way of giving radiotherapy, called brachytherapy, which involves putting small radioactive seeds into the prostate, so that the radiotherapy is given from inside the gland. Each seed irradiates a very small amount of tissue immediately around it. This means that a lot of seeds have to be used, and they need placing with care. The advantage is that even with seeds put very close to the surface of the prostate, the radiation is virtually confined to it, protecting the rectum and the bladder.

This is not a particularly new idea – some years ago the seeds were put into the prostate after the surgeon had exposed it through a surgical incision. Now, a urologist or oncologist can use a transrectal ultrasound probe (see page 83) to help see where to place the seeds. The seeds are inserted via needles put into the prostate (under an anaesthetic) through the skin just in front of the back passage. It can be done as a day-case procedure.

This method certainly produces few side effects in most patients (although very rarely it can cause severe pain or difficulty passing urine). At present it looks as if it is a good way of getting rid of the cancer, but it has not been around as long as ordinary radiotherapy or radical prostatectomy. It probably will be some years before we can really be sure how it compares with these other treatments.

Brachytherapy on its own is suitable only for smaller tumours confined to inside of the prostate, but is sometimes used in combination with external radiotherapy for more advanced cancer. Brachytherapy is becoming more commonly used.

Active surveillance

As many tumours are not immediately dangerous, some patients may be advised that they need no immediate treatment. This is called 'watchful waiting' or 'active surveillance'. It does not mean that they are being neglected, and it is important that they are seen regularly, so that tests can be done to check that the cancer is not advancing. If it is, treatment might then be advised.

Although we are still not very good at predicting how rapidly a cancer will grow, its appearance under the microscope (see 'Gleason score' on page 69) may help. Sometimes the tests will show that the tumour is growing so slowly that it is safe to discharge the patient from the hospital clinic, although he will be advised to keep in touch with his GP.

Also, as early prostate cancer is unlikely to get rapidly out of control, some urologists recommend a few months of observation. By measuring how quickly the level of PSA is increasing (if at all), they can identify the type of cancer that does require treatment.

Choice of treatment

If treatment is recommended for cancer when it is at an early stage, and confined to the prostate gland, a discussion will usually take place about the choice of treatment. As the best treatment for early cancer of the prostate is uncertain, a man with the disease should expect to be informed of the possibilities and given a major say in deciding what is done.

What is involved in radical prostatectomy?

Radical prostatectomy involves removal of the whole prostate gland. This is different from operations for BPH, where even the open operation takes out only the inner enlarged part of the gland. The prostate gland can be removed either through an incision in the lower abdomen or from below by an incision in front of the back passage.

Either before or at the same time (possibly by a laparoscopic 'keyhole' operation) the lymph nodes (glands) at the side of the prostate will be removed and checked to make sure that there is no sign of the cancer spreading. Removal of these nodes causes no harm. If there is no cancer in them, the prostate gland is removed, cutting the urethra below the prostate and removing the prostate from the neck of the bladder, which is then stitched back onto the urethra.

A catheter is left in place, usually for two weeks while healing takes place. Most men get over the immediate effects of the operation quickly enough to go home after a few days with the catheter in, returning to hospital to have it removed.

Complications of radical prostatectomy

The biggest problem during the operation is a risk of bleeding from large veins in front of the prostate – a blood transfusion sometimes is necessary if this happens. A little urine may leak from where the bladder is stitched to the urethra but this usually settles down. The two problems which can be found afterwards are poor control of the urine and sexual difficulties.

Poor control of urine

In an earlier chapter, the closeness of the muscle sphincters of the bladder and the prostate was described. Removing the prostate can affect these muscles. It is quite common to have some difficulty in control of urine for a day or two after the catheter is removed.

The patient will be warned of this and taught exercises to strengthen his muscles. Although most men regain control very quickly, some find that they are left with a little leakage from time to time – for example, during exercise or in bed at night – and they may sometimes need to wear a pad for protection.

Very occasionally the leakage of urine is more serious. If treatment is needed, a plastic device called an artificial sphincter might be put in by another operation, but this is unusual.

Sexual problems

The nerves needed for a man to have an erection lie close to his prostate. At one time it was thought that a radical prostatectomy almost inevitably caused a loss of erection because these nerves were cut. Surgeons now know more precisely where the nerves are, and the operation is done in such a way that damage to them is avoided if possible. However, the surgeon will warn the patient that cutting these nerves is still sometimes necessary to remove the cancer completely.

As nerves are easily bruised but can recover, an initial loss of erection may improve but can take many months. It is only the actual erection that is affected – normal sexual desire and ability to reach a climax and orgasm should not be affected, although there will be little in the way of fluid (ejaculate) to come out.

If the nerves are only partially damaged, one of the new oral erectile dysfunction treatments may help. If the nerves are cut completely, treatment is still possible, but the patient will need to learn to use injections given into the penis.

What is involved in radiotherapy?
External beam radiotherapy

Radiotherapy is given by a machine under which the patient lies for a few minutes for each treatment. A number of daily treatments (called fractions) are usually given spread over four to six weeks. Patients normally have radiotherapy as outpatients, although in some cases admission to hospital is advised.

The period of treatment with, and time to get over, radiotherapy is very similar to the time it takes to recover after a radical prostatectomy. Usually either treatment means taking a couple of months off work.

Complications

It is unusual for radiotherapy to cause incontinence of urine and, although failure of erection occurs quite often, it is less common than after radical prostatectomy. However, because it is impossible to focus the radiotherapy entirely on the prostate, it does also temporarily affect the bladder and the rectum (back passage).

Most men will get some symptoms of cystitis (burning and frequent passage of urine) and diarrhoea during and after radiotherapy. Sometimes blood will be seen in the urine or bowel motions.

These symptoms usually settle down within a few weeks of completing treatment. Occasionally symptoms will persist and, very rarely, the radiotherapy might produce some permanent damage to the bladder or bowel.

Conformal radiotherapy

A new type of radiotherapy is now being introduced called 'conformal radiotherapy'. This enables the radiation to be concentrated on the tumour itself, reducing the exposure of the surrounding tissues. This should reduce the risk of side effects, but in addition can be used to increase the amount of radiation given to the actual tumour, possibly increasing its effectiveness.

Brachytherapy

Before it can be decided whether brachytherapy is possible, a careful assessment is needed. Only small tumours confined to the prostate are considered suitable. It is also difficult to put the seeds in properly if the prostate is very large. Sometimes it is possible to give hormone treatment for two to three months first to reduce the prostate to a suitable size.

Brachytherapy

Brachytherapy involves placing small radioactive 'seeds' into the prostate, so that radiotherapy is given from inside the gland.

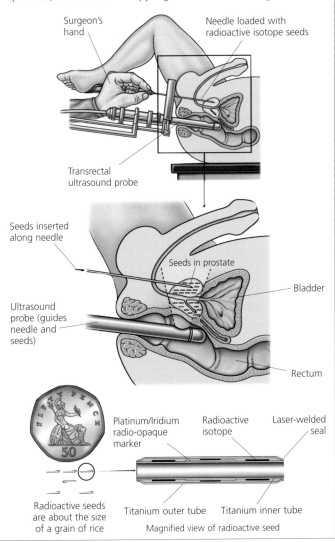

Surgeon's hand

Needle loaded with radioactive isotope seeds

Transrectal ultrasound probe

Seeds inserted along needle

Seeds in prostate

Bladder

Ultrasound probe (guides needle and seeds)

Rectum

Platinum/Iridium radio-opaque marker

Radioactive isotope

Laser-welded seal

Radioactive seeds are about the size of a grain of rice

Titanium outer tube

Titanium inner tube

Magnified view of radioactive seed

The prostate tends to swell and, if there is already some blockage to the urethra by the prostate, this might increase causing problems passing urine. Usually a flow rate measurement (see page 31) will be done and, if it is severely reduced, the patient is advised that brachytherapy is not for him. A previous TURP (see page 41) will distort the prostate, and certainly if this operation has been done recently it makes brachytherapy unwise.

If all these problems are avoided and it is decided to go ahead, it is done in two stages. The patient has a very careful transrectal ultrasound scan, which is used to plan how many seeds are needed, and to make a sort of map to show where they are to be put.

The actual operation is done at a second session, usually a week or two later. Under an anaesthetic, a series of needles is pushed into the prostate from below using the 'map'.

The seeds are joined together in strands, and a length of strand containing the right number of seeds is passed into each needle, after which it is withdrawn leaving the seeds in the right bit of the prostate. A catheter may be used for a day or two to drain urine from the bladder, but once the patient has recovered from the anaesthetic he should be able to go home.

Not only is the actual procedure complicated, but it has to be done in a centre with the facilities and specially trained physicists to calculate the dose of seeds. Until recently brachytherapy was done only in very few places, but the number of centres has increased. Now most men should be able to get the treatment, although they may still have to travel further to have it done than they would for ordinary radiotherapy or surgery.

Cryotherapy

As with brachytherapy, this is not a particularly new idea. It consists of using a special probe that literally freezes the prostate. As with brachytherapy, improvements in technology have made the treatment more effective by enabling it to be better localised to the prostate. In the past there was quite a risk of damaging surrounding organs.

As with many new treatments, it requires expensive equipment. This treatment is being tested in a number of places, mainly in the USA and, even if these tests give promising results, it is unlikely that it will be widely available in this country for some time. It might turn out to be a useful treatment if the cancer in the prostate starts to grow again after radiotherapy.

Which treatment is best?

Surprisingly, there is still no agreement among doctors as to which is the best treatment for early prostate cancer, or indeed whether surgery or radiotherapy is any better than simply keeping a close eye on the disease and treating it only if it starts to advance ('active surveillance').

Why do opinions differ?

This is because, even when the disease is in an active form, it will still usually develop slowly, and may take many years to become serious. Also, with better methods of diagnosis, tumours are being picked up that are very unlikely to be harmful. As many men with prostate cancer are quite old, they often will have, or will soon develop, other illnesses that might be more dangerous.

This issue is much debated and, although a lot of information is available, it is difficult to compare different treatments because they are not always used in similar circumstances. For example, someone who is less physically fit is more likely to be treated with radiotherapy than by an operation. This will produce a bias – that is, if there is a difference in outcome it may be the result of differences in the type of patient treated, rather than one treatment being better than another.

Clinical trials

To investigate this type of problem really requires a randomised trial (see page 108). The results of a trial in Scandinavia comparing radical prostatectomy with watchful waiting ('active surveillance') were recently published. At this stage, in the group who had the operation, half as many men have died from prostate cancer compared with the other group.

This looks good for the operation, but it is not as simple as that. In both groups only a small number of patients have died from prostate cancer, with many more dying from other diseases. This means that, although the operation was beneficial for a few men, there were many more who did not benefit because the prostate cancer developed so slowly that it did not endanger their lives.

As a result of this, most experts feel that the question has not yet been answered, and the results of other trials in progress will be important. In one of these, which is taking place in Britain, men are being invited to have a PSA test (see page 60) and if, as a result, they are found to have cancer, they are invited to be randomised to have radical prostatectomy, radiotherapy or surveillance. This study hopes to collect a large number of patients and should provide a lot of information. Other studies of treatment in the USA, and of screening with PSA in Europe and the USA, might within the next 10 years enable us to give clearer advice on what is the best treatment.

Personal choice

Meanwhile, it is really a case of the patient's priorities. There can be little doubt that some (but possibly only a minority of) men will be cured by treatment, but for many more the treatment may be unnecessary. Some men will want to take this chance, whereas others may be prepared to take the risk of a shorter lifespan to avoid the immediate risks and side effects of the treatment.

There can at present be no simple piece of advice that applies to everyone. Some men are happier with an operation, knowing that it aims to remove the cancer completely from the body. Others do not like operations and prefer radiotherapy, which would also be suggested to someone who was not particularly fit for an operation. For someone who had other serious illnesses, active surveillance would be strongly recommended.

Preliminary hormone treatment

Sometimes, before radical prostatectomy or radiotherapy, a temporary period of hormone treatment (see page 88) is given to reduce the size of the prostate. This is thought to improve the effectiveness of the treatment and is more often done before radiotherapy treatment rather than radical prostatectomy.

During this treatment, which is usually given for three months or a little longer, the side effects of hormone treatment are experienced but, once the radiotherapy (or operation) has been completed, the hormone treatment is stopped and its effects should be reversed. Sometimes, if the tumour in the prostate is particularly large, a combination of radiotherapy and hormone treatment, continuing after the radiotherapy has finished, is recommended.

Advanced prostatic cancer

Unfortunately, when tests are done after cancer has been diagnosed, they may show that it is too advanced to be permanently cured by surgery or radiotherapy. Sometimes after initially successful treatment with surgery or radiotherapy, tests show that the cancer has recurred.

However, this is far from being a hopeless situation. In the first place, the tumour may only be slow growing and elderly men with the disease may not have their lives shortened because of it. However, when prostatic cancer is more active, there is much that can be done to relieve symptoms and to slow its growth.

In addition to the usual prostatic symptoms, advanced prostatic cancer can cause backache (probably the most common effect) or pain in other bones, general ill health with loss of weight, anaemia and other problems. Weakening of the bones can result in fractures, but this is not common. Occasionally, cancer in the prostate can block the drainage of the kidneys. All these problems can improve, often almost completely, after treatment.

Hormone treatment

Over 50 years ago an American urologist called Charles Huggins found that, if he removed the testicles from dogs with prostatic cancer, their cancer got smaller (regressed).

Hormone control of prostate growth

The growth of the prostate gland is controlled largely by the male sex hormone, testosterone. It is produced in the testicles in response to signals from the pituitary gland in the brain.

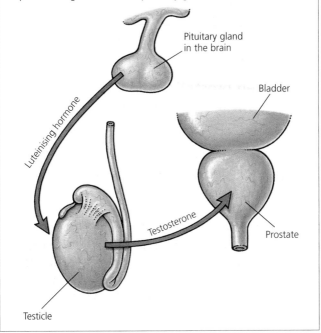

Pituitary gland in the brain

Bladder

Luteinising hormone

Testosterone

Prostate

Testicle

He then treated some men by the same operation and some by giving them female hormones, and he found that their disease responded in the same way.

This was one of the earliest examples of an effective treatment for cancer that had spread beyond surgical cure. It was so important that Huggins was given the Nobel Prize for Medicine.

Hormone treatment is still the most effective way of treating advanced cancer of the prostate, although there are now new ways of doing it.

The prostate will only grow and work if it receives normal amounts of male hormones (androgens). There are a number of different androgens of which the most important is testosterone. Cancer of the prostate cannot grow without androgens, so depriving it of these hormones causes it to shrink and sometimes to disappear. Testosterone is produced from the testicles in response to a hormone which comes from a small gland at the base of the brain (the pituitary).

As doctors and scientists have come to understand this, so new methods of hormone treatment have been developed. We now have much more choice than Dr Huggins had back in the 1940s. The testicles can be prevented from producing the hormone, either by an operation to remove their functioning part (or sometimes the whole testicle is removed) or by drugs.

Alternatively, there are drugs that act as a barrier between the tumour and the androgens. These drugs prevent the androgens from stimulating the tumour cells without reducing the amount of androgen in the blood.

Choice of treatment

Generally speaking, the effect of these different treatments on the tumour is the same. The choice between them is made on the basis of how they are given and of their possible side effects. Also, if one treatment doesn't suit an individual patient, it can be changed to another one.

As with deciding between surgery and radiotherapy for early cancer, the patient may well be asked his opinion and therefore it is useful here to give a little more information about the possibilities. As far as the patient is concerned, he can have:

- an operation that gets the whole thing over with so he no longer has to worry about taking treatment
- an injection once a month or every three months
- tablets.

As the hormone or drug treatments work only while they are being given, injections or tablets have to be taken indefinitely.

Treatment by operation

The usual operation is called a subcapsular orchiectomy and involves making a cut into each of the testicles and removing the active tissue from the inside so they no longer produce testosterone. Occasionally, removal of the whole testicle might be recommended.

Treatment by injection

The injections are of a type of drug called a luteinising hormone-releasing hormone analogue (LHRH analogue) – for example, goserelin (Zoladex), leuprorelin (Prostap SR) or triptorelin (Decapeptyl SR). These injections stop the testicles producing testosterone and the effects are very similar to the operation.

These injections originally had to be given once a month, but types are now available that can last for three months or longer. Even longer periods may be possible in future. Although longer-acting injections contain a larger amount of the drug, this does not mean that they have a 'stronger effect' – the drug is released slowly. This means that the effect is the same but the drug is present for a longer time before it needs replacing with another injection. It is simply a matter of the convenience of having fewer injections. If you have been having injections once a month and

Subcapsular orchiectomy to treat prostate cancer

A cut is made into each testicle and the active tissue is removed. The testes no longer produce testosterone and the prostate cancer cannot grow without it.

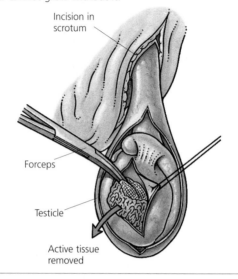

Incision in scrotum

Forceps

Testicle

Active tissue removed

are happy with this, there is no reason to change – the effects on the cancer are just the same.

Side effects from operation or injections

Whether the treatment is an operation, or an injection given monthly, three monthly or longer, the level of male hormone is reduced.

Sexual activity

Most men find that, as a result, their sexual activity – both their desire for sex and their ability to have an erection – is lost. Very occasionally this does not happen, for reasons that are not understood; this should be thought of as a bonus and it does not mean that the treatment will not be effective.

Hot flushes

Hot flushes, very similar to the condition experienced by women during the menopause, are another problem. These consist of feeling hot, or of attacks of sweating. Although fairly common, most men are only mildly affected and the condition tends to improve. If hot flushes are more severe, treatment is available. It is important to realise that they are a side effect of the treatment – some men worry that hot flushes might be a sign that the cancer is advancing.

Smaller testicles

The effect of the operation on the testicles is to reduce their size, but the injection treatment also causes shrinkage. The testicles are associated with masculinity and it is natural to feel that this type of treatment involves 'castration'. However, most men with advanced prostatic cancer feel so much better as the treatment starts to work that this does not usually worry them too much.

Weight gain and bone weakness

However, the loss of the 'male drive' from testosterone does, in some cases, cause tiredness and lassitude. Some men also put on weight and there is evidence that this weight increase can be at the expense of a reduction in the amount of body muscle. Slightly more worrying is the fact that, in the long term, loss of testosterone may cause some weakness or thinning of the bones, as occurs in women after the menopause.

Generally speaking, in a man with advanced prostatic cancer, the benefits of the treatment far outweigh these possible side effects. The doctor advising on the treatment will have these side effects in mind and, because of them, it is sometimes recommended that treatment is delayed until it is really necessary.

Pros and cons of both treatments

Although the operation and the injections have very similar effects in the long run, there are differences between them at the time the treatment is started.

Orchiectomy is only a fairly minor operation, but it does mean going into hospital, usually requires a general anaesthetic and is painful for several days. Minor complications such as bruising or swelling, or wound infection, are not unusual.

The operation works straight away and sometimes the symptoms are better as soon as the patient wakes up from the anaesthetic.

The injections work more slowly, and in fact during the first few weeks of treatment they actually cause an increase in the amount of testosterone. This could make the cancer grow a little. Often, for this reason, tablets of another type of hormone treatment are also given for a few weeks, starting several days before the first injection.

Treatment given as tablets

This may be prescribed because the patient prefers this type of medicine. Also, if the patient really wishes to avoid loss of sexual function, there is a type of drug called an anti-androgen.

Anti-androgens

These prevent the action of the testosterone on the tumour without reducing its level in the blood, and this can preserve sexual function. There are several of this type of drug available including:

- flutamide (Drogenil)
- bicalutamide (Casodex).

Flutamide (Drogenil) has been available for some time – it did tend to have more side effects than other forms of treatment, including gastrointestinal upset. Bicalutamide (Casodex) has been introduced more recently and may have fewer side effects.

Another drug called cyproterone acetate (Cyprostat) is also quite frequently prescribed. As well as blocking the effects of testosterone on the prostate, because it is similar to a type of female hormone, cyproterone acetate also reduces testosterone levels. Until recently, six tablets had to be taken each day, but now a larger tablet is available. Very rarely it can cause damage to the liver and, as with all these treatments, must be carefully supervised.

Female hormones

At one time female oestrogen hormones such as diethylstilbestrol were used a lot to treat cancer of the prostate. However, they cause swelling of the breasts, but perhaps more importantly can have serious effects on the heart. Although they can be used safely in very small doses, most men who are treated with tablets are given one of the other types of drug.

There are other ways of giving hormone treatment, and newer and possibly better ones are being developed. However, the treatments mentioned here are the most common ones.

Combining drugs

Recently it was found that a greater reduction of male hormone is possible by using a combination of drugs. This is because the adrenal glands also make male hormones and are not affected by orchiectomy or LHRH analogues.

Whether this more intense treatment actually improves results has been much debated by specialists. There is some evidence that it does, at least in some circumstances, and some patients receive it. Unfortunately it is more complicated and can cause more side effects.

What if the cancer has spread?
Radiotherapy

If the cancer has spread to bone and is causing pain, radiotherapy can be very effective and usually works quickly. Sometimes a course of treatments – usually ten – is given, either as an outpatient or as an inpatient. Sometimes only a single treatment is necessary. Usually there are few problems but, depending where the painful area is, a mild stomach or bowel upset might occur.

Another method of giving radiotherapy to the bone is to use a radioactive substance called strontium-89 (Metastron). This selects out the parts of the bone where the cancer is and gives it very intense but localised and safe radiation. It is given as an outpatient by a simple injection, so is very easy, although some simple precautions about radiation are needed for a day or two. Although strontium-89 is the most common isotope used for this purpose, others are being introduced.

Note that it was strontium-90 that used to cause all the concern about radioactive fallout – strontium-89 is a completely different type of strontium as far as its radiation is concerned and does not have the same harmful effects.

Chemotherapy

Until recently, anti-cancer drugs did not seem to be very effective against prostate cancer, and many patients were elderly and often too unwell to tolerate the side effects. However, chemotherapy is now used more often, mainly in patients in whom the effect of hormone therapy is beginning to wear off.

Part of the reason is that the prostate-specific antigen or PSA test (see page 60) helps doctors to diagnose relapse of the disease at an earlier stage, and the treatment can be started when it is likely to be most effective and the patient still well enough to cope with it. The other reason is that in clinical trials some of the newer drugs have been effective and well tolerated.

A drug called docetaxel, in particular, has been shown to help symptoms and to prolong life in men with advanced disease. Usually given along with a hormone treatment, it is likely that this and other chemotherapy drugs will be used increasingly in treating men with prostate cancer.

Bisphosphonates

Many of the problems with advanced prostate cancer

come from metastases in the bones, which can be painful and cause the bones to break or collapse. Bisphosphonates are a type of drug developed originally to treat other bone diseases such as osteoporosis. They have also been shown to relieve pain and prevent other problems from bone metastases, including those from prostate cancer. Some of them (for example, pamidronate) are taken as tablets, but a newer and probably the most effective one, zoledronate, is given by infusion into a vein every three weeks.

New and future treatments for prostate cancer

A lot of research into the reasons why cells become cancerous is leading to treatments that interfere with the cancer process, some of which may be introduced soon. It must be emphasised that, although these treatments are effective, they are not dramatic breakthroughs and will not replace the conventional treatments described earlier in this chapter. However, the new treatments will help men in whom treatment has not been successful, or where the effects of treatment are wearing off.

Gene therapy

Promising future developments include gene therapy in which the genetics of the cancer cell is changed. This type of treatment might be used to repair damage to the gene that is producing the cancer, to introduce genes or related molecules that kill the cells or stop them growing, or to make the cells more susceptible to drugs or other substances that will destroy them.

Prostate cancer may be a particularly good form of the disease for these treatments, because some of them need to be injected directly into the tumour, which is easy to do in the prostate (see 'Radiotherapy – brachytherapy', page 76).

Immunotherapy
Another promising approach is immunotherapy where antibodies or immune cells are produced against the tumour cells.

Prevention of prostate cancer
Although treatment of cancer is improving, it would be better to prevent it in the first place. The best example of cancer prevention is stopping smoking to reduce the risk of getting lung cancer. It is possible that ways of preventing prostate cancer will soon be found.

Nutrition
Although Japanese men are much less prone to prostate cancer than westerners, if they move from Japan to the USA, their risk of getting the disease increases. This is thought to have something to do with diet. A diet high in animal fat may increase the risk of prostate cancer, whereas some vitamins and other substances may have a protective effect. More importantly, soy products in the Japanese diet may act like a mild female hormone (called a phytoestrogen).

Drugs
Finasteride, a drug used to treat benign prostatic hyperplasia (see page 14), reduces the activity of male hormone within the prostate, and so could influence the development of prostate cancer. A study in which 18,000 men took either finasteride or a placebo for seven years has recently reported its results. The number

who developed cancer was reduced by a quarter in the men who took finasteride.

However, this reduction was in the number of very early tumours detected when the patients' prostates were biopsied, and it is not clear how much this would affect the number of men who will actually develop symptoms or die from prostate cancer. There was also some concern that, although the total number of prostate cancers was less, the number with so-called high-grade tumours (see 'Gleason score', page 69), which are the more dangerous ones, may have increased in those taking finasteride.

The importance of these results is not too clear, but it is certainly too early to recommend that finasteride is used as a preventive treatment. Nor should men already taking the drug worry that it is likely to be doing any harm.

Other substances
Trials using other substances that might prevent prostate cancer are going on at present.

KEY POINTS

■ Prostatic cancer may be treated by surgery, radiotherapy or hormone therapy

■ Removing the whole prostate (radical prostatectomy) is possible when the cancer is only inside the prostate

■ Radiotherapy is an alternative to radical prostatectomy and can treat a tumour too advanced for surgery

■ Hormone treatment is useful for advanced prostatic disease

Prostatitis and chronic pelvic pain syndrome

Acute prostatitis
Symptoms
Inflammation of the prostate can occur at almost any age. It is often caused by infection. Although cystitis – an infection of the bladder causing burning and frequency – is a disease that more commonly affects women, if it occurs in a man it often causes an infection of the prostate called acute prostatitis.

This can make the patient very unwell with a high temperature and other symptoms. In an older man who also has benign prostatic hyperplasia (BPH), any prostate symptoms might become worse, and sometimes prostatitis can cause retention of urine. In addition, sometimes an infection of the testicle called epididymitis complicates prostatitis and the symptoms from this might overshadow those from the prostate itself.

Treatment

As with simple cystitis, prostatitis is treated with antibiotics. However, the prostate does not take up antibiotics very well and some antibiotics don't work properly inside the prostate. If an infection of the prostate is suspected, the most likely type of antibiotic to be used is called a quinolone – examples are ciprofloxacin (Ciproxin), ofloxacin (Tarivid) and norfloxacin (Utinor).

It is important that the antibiotic be used for long enough to get rid of the infection completely. This usually means several weeks of treatment. It is also important that the full course of antibiotics be taken, even if the symptoms have gone completely, to prevent the infection flaring up again.

Taking plenty of fluids (sometimes an intravenous drip is needed) and rest is important while the symptoms are bad. Avoiding sex is probably wise, but most patients won't feel like it anyway while the symptoms are bad! Afterwards, frequent sex might help, as every time a climax is reached the fluid from the prostate may flush out any remaining infection.

Rarely an abscess might develop. This is treated by letting out the pus via an operation very similar to a transurethral resection of the prostate (TURP).

Chronic pelvic pain syndrome

Symptoms

A chronic infection in the prostate can lead to occasional flare-ups of cystitis-like symptoms or cause more chronic pain. The pain occurs in the lower abdomen, the testicles, between the legs or even in the back passage. However, similar symptoms can occur in the absence of infection. As the word prostatitis implies infection, or at least inflammation, in the prostate, most urologists now prefer to describe conditions causing these symptoms as 'chronic pelvic pain'.

Treatment

Diagnosing an actual infection in the prostate can be very difficult. The prostate may be tender on examination. The doctor may try to grow bacteria from the prostatic fluid, which can be obtained by massaging the prostate or by getting a sample of semen.

Often, treatment with a four- to six-week course of one of the antibiotics named above is tried. If this has no effect, it probably means that an infection is not the cause of the problem.

Sometimes the prostate is inflamed, but doesn't seem to be infected by bacteria. The cause of this is not really understood but the symptoms are sometimes helped by anti-inflammatory drugs such as ibuprofen (Brufen, Nurofen) or indometacin (Indocid) – although many similar drugs might be used.

Prostatodynia

However, the same symptoms can occur without even inflammation, a condition that used to be called prostatodynia. This may result from spasm of the muscle in the prostate. Certainly many men who suffer from it are helped by relaxing this muscle, with the same alpha-blocker drugs used to treat symptoms from BPH (see page 49).

Reassurance and regular checks

These conditions can be among the most difficult to treat. When they recur repeatedly, they can be very debilitating for the patient and cause a lot of anxiety, which in itself can aggravate the symptoms.

In such cases it is very helpful to have the prostate checked out and for the man to be reassured that there is nothing else wrong with it. However, it must be emphasised that it is very unusual for pain in the prostate to be caused by cancer.

Also, because the symptoms are not very specific, if the urologist finds nothing wrong the man may be referred to another specialist to make sure that there is not another cause for them. Some men find regular contact with a specialist, mainly for reassurance and counselling, helpful.

In severe cases treatment in a specialised pain clinic can be helpful.

Asymptomatic prostatic infection

Infection in the prostate does not always cause symptoms. Some men who suffer from repeated urinary infections, despite their being well between attacks, have a chronic infection. Short courses of treatment deal with the symptoms, but do not get rid of the infection completely, so it flares up again in a few weeks or months.

Treatment

Again, the solution is a long course of one of the antibiotics mentioned earlier. If you are ever in this situation, it is important to take the whole course of treatment even if the symptoms resolve long before it has been completed.

Raised PSA

Asymptomatic infection can cause another problem, because it is one of the conditions other than cancer that can increase the level of PSA (see page 60). If a man has a raised PSA and it is thought unlikely that he has cancer, he may be prescribed a course of antibiotics to see if this brings the PSA down to a normal level.

Much has still to be learnt about this range of conditions, which have perhaps been neglected in the past. They are now subject to increasing research and it is hoped that treatment for the many men who have intractable symptoms will improve in future.

KEY POINTS

- Inflammation of the prostate (chronic pelvic pain) may be caused by infection
- Treatment is usually with antibiotics

Improving treatment

How is treatment being improved?

This book makes it clear that there have been many new developments in managing prostate disorders. As benign prostatic hyperplasia (BPH) is so common, it would be a major step forward in improving men's health if we could find a way of preventing it. In fact, it is probably possible to do this already.

From the way it works, the prostate drugs, finasteride and dutasteride, might be better at preventing BPH than treating it once it has occurred. Unfortunately, all men would have to start taking it when they reach 40 and continue every day for the rest of their lives. For a disease that in most cases is a nuisance rather than life threatening, this is not practical, nor could our overstretched National Health Service afford it.

As new, more effective drugs are found, and technology such as thermotherapy and laser devices is improved, the day may come when TURP and other 'old-fashioned' prostate operations are no longer done.

Cancer of the prostate is a very important disease. If treatments were simpler and easier than removing the prostate or radiotherapy, it would be much more feasible to tackle it by screening to look for early disease. We are beginning to know a little more about causes of prostate cancer. Although we can diagnose cancer at an early stage, many of the cancers diagnosed develop very slowly and may not be that dangerous.

If the cancers that were dangerous could be identified, treatment could be concentrated on the patients with these, and we could avoid other patients having to undergo treatments from which they may not benefit, and which might do them more harm than good. We are beginning to know a little more about the causes of prostate cancer and, as described on page 98, we might be able to find ways of preventing it.

Clinical trials

Many new methods of treatment for both BPH and cancer are being tried at present. Such treatments can be tested only with the help of people with the disease. These are called clinical trials and are an essential part of showing that a new treatment really does work and that it is safe.

If you have a prostate condition you might be asked to take part in a clinical trial. Usually, this will be for some treatment that has already been extensively tested, so is almost certainly safe and there is a good chance it will be helpful. Indeed, sometimes being in a clinical trial is the only way to be treated with a promising new drug.

Double-blind trials

Most trials are of a type called double-blind randomised studies. These either compare two different treatments or one treatment against an inactive dummy treatment called a placebo. The comparison is only worthwhile if the treatment taken is chosen by chance or randomisation. So that the interpretation of the results is done fairly, neither the patients nor the doctors running the trial know which of the treatments each patient is taking – although, if for some reason they need to know, they can easily find out.

Placebo effect

Why is a placebo necessary? Simply seeing a doctor and getting any attention tends to make you feel better. This placebo effect is seen a lot in trials in BPH. This may be because the attention that patients receive makes them less bothered about their disease, and one result of this is that the muscle in the prostate relaxes. Patients receiving only inactive placebo may not only notice fewer symptoms, but their flow rate may also improve, so it is very important to compare drugs with a placebo to make sure that it really is the drug that is making things better.

Taking part in a trial

If you do take part in a trial, you will certainly receive a lot of attention and many patients appreciate this. On the other hand, it does also mean attending the hospital much more often and some people find this difficult. The main disadvantage in most trials is that you have to have a lot of blood samples taken – if you can't stand needles, trials aren't for you.

Before a trial is allowed to take place in any hospital, it will have been carefully considered by either a regional, or the hospital's own, ethical committee to make sure that it is safe and sensible. You will be given a very full explanation, both verbally by a doctor and in writing, and it will be entirely your choice whether you take part.

You should not take part simply to please the doctor. No one will object if you don't accept an invitation to join a trial and you will still get all the treatment that you need.

Who will treat you?

Many diseases are treated by both hospital specialists and GPs, sometimes jointly. Patients with diabetes and high blood pressure will be used to this.

Until recently, the only real treatment for BPH, the most common disease of the prostate, was an operation. This meant referral to a hospital urologist and it was not worthwhile for GPs to get too involved – there were too many other calls on their time.

Unless the GP decided the problem was so mild that no treatment was going to be needed, a referral to a urologist was obviously the best thing for the patient. Even now most men with prostate problems will be seen and investigated in a urology clinic.

However, the treatment of prostate disorders has changed now that there are drugs that can be prescribed for BPH. Men with prostate symptoms are now less likely to put up with them than they were. People are living longer so there are far more men around who are old enough to have prostate trouble than there used to be.

Milder forms of BPH can be managed with drugs, so it is no longer absolutely necessary for a surgical specialist such as a urologist to treat every patient. However, it is important that the patient and his prostate are carefully looked at before starting treatment, both to make sure that drugs are the right thing and to rule out cancer or other serious conditions that do need to be treated by a urologist.

Some GPs have become very enthusiastic about this and a few health centres are now equipped with urine flow machines so that most of the important tests can be done by the GP. More often, the GP wants to know about the tests but can't do them all.

Open access clinics

Some hospitals have set up 'open access BPH clinics' where the patient can go for the tests without having to be seen by a consultant urologist. As described under 'Having the prostate investigated' (page 25), many of these clinics are now staffed by specially trained nurses who, in a lot of cases, also do the rectal examination of the prostate.

The results of the tests are sent to the GP, but will also be looked at in the hospital and usually some advice is given. Any evidence of cancer will be picked up and the patient would then be seen promptly by the urologist in charge of the clinic.

This system has many advantages for the patient:

- He will almost certainly be seen quicker – most clinics offer appointments within a month or less.

- In a clinic where only men with prostate disease are seen, everything will be done more efficiently.

- The staff are all knowledgeable about the particular problem and may have more time to give information and to answer questions.

- Many men are more comfortable having a somewhat embarrassing problem dealt with in close consultation with a GP whom they have known for years than they are seeing a strange hospital specialist.

It is difficult to predict the future, but large health centres could start to run their own clinics. This can be done either with a visiting hospital urologist or perhaps with one of the partners in the practice specialising – not only in managing BPH but also in managing other urinary diseases.

Patients should be reassured that these changes can only improve the care of men with BPH and they reflect the increased awareness of this condition in recent years.

KEY POINTS

■ Determined efforts are being made to find better treatments for prostate disorders

■ Clinical trials are essential to show that a treatment really does work and is safe

■ New open access clinics are being set up to improve the care of men with prostate problems

Questions and answers

Why does benign prostatic hyperplasia (BPH) and cancer of the prostate occur only in older men?
Some growth of the prostate probably occurs throughout adult life, under the influence of male hormones. About the age of 50, changes take place in the way the body produces and deals with male hormones, and this seems to cause the more rapid growth that is BPH. These hormone changes might influence cancer of the prostate, but many other types of cancer also occur more commonly in older people. This is probably because whatever causes the cancer takes many years to have an effect.

Why doesn't everybody with BPH get symptoms from it?
We don't quite understand this. Certainly, a small prostate can cause very bad symptoms, while men with huge prostates can have virtually no trouble. It probably depends partly on just how the prostate squeezes the urethra and how well the bladder can cope with any obstruction. Anyway, it's all relative. Probably

there are very few elderly men who aren't a little bit affected, but many have symptoms so mild and that develop so slowly that they don't really notice them.

Can disease from the prostate cause illness in sexual partners?

No. BPH is specific to the prostate so can't occur in females, and in any case it is not caused by anything that could be transmitted in this way. The same applies to prostatic cancer. Although it is possible for the prostate to be affected by sexually transmitted infections, this is unusual, and prostatitis does not carry any risk to the patient's partner, nor is it caught by sexual contact.

I sometimes see blood in my semen – is this a sign of prostate disease?

Blood in the semen is quite common, although for obvious reasons it might not always be noticed. Unlike blood in the urine it is rarely a sign of serious illness. It can be compared to a nose bleed. Like nose bleeds it can sometimes occur repeatedly for a short period of time then settle down. Just as most nose bleeds are harmless, so is blood in the semen.

Very rarely, they can both be a sign of a disease affecting the blood, or something like high blood pressure, or can result from some local disease that causes bleeding. Occasionally, blood in the semen is associated with small stones in the prostate and it can sometimes complicate prostatitis. Although BPH and prostate cancer can cause bleeding, this is usually seen in the urine.

Blood in the semen is not usually something to worry about but, if it recurs it is important to have it checked out.

Can I do anything to reduce the risk of prostate disease?
There is probably not a lot you can do to prevent BPH.
However, if you have a bit of trouble, it is possible to stop
it getting worse by being sensible.

It is important to drink enough. Spread your
drinking evenly through the day – if you are liable to
wake at night, cut down a little in the evening and
don't drink a lot of tea, coffee or beer just before
going to bed.

Avoid hanging on too long, make a point of passing
urine regularly at comfortable intervals. On the other
hand, if you do find that you are getting a bit of
frequency, don't let it take over – it is easy to get into
the habit of passing urine more often than you really
need to and this just makes things worse.

With regard to prostatic cancer, a number of trials
of various measures, including drug treatment, are
under way to see whether prostate cancer can be
prevented. We are also beginning to understand how
diet can affect the risk of developing prostate cancer.
It does seem as though fatty foods will increase the
risk. Some forms of vegetables, including tomatoes
and soya products, seem to have a protective effect.

In general, a 'healthy diet' – plenty of fruit and
vegetables, not too much fat or meat – as well as being
good for your general health may reduce the risk of
getting prostate cancer. As prostate cancer may take
many years to develop, it is probably a case of the
earlier this is done, the better. There is more about
prevention on page 99.

I've just had prostatitis. Does this mean that I'm likely
to get prostate trouble when I'm an old man?
Not really. Prostatitis doesn't cause either BPH or

cancer. Of course, prostate trouble is common, so you might be going to get it anyway.

I sometimes have pain in my testicles. Is this caused by prostate disease?

Pain in the testicles is a very common symptom. Usually no cause can be found for it and it settles down without treatment. However, if you have any concerns or unusual symptoms, consult your doctor promptly. At the best of times, the testicles are a bit sensitive, and sometimes this sensitivity seems to increase for a while for some reason:

- Discomfort occurs from time to time in men who have had vasectomy operations.

- As the tubes from the testicles go into the prostate, it is possible for infection to spread down them.

- Very painful swelling of the epididymis, which is attached to the back of the testicle, called epididymitis, sometimes occurs in men with BPH or during an attack of prostatitis.

- If a hard lump is felt in the testicle itself, it could be a tumour and should be reported to your doctor straight away.

My father died from cancer of the prostate. Is the same thing likely to happen to me?

Not necessarily. However, there seems to be a type of prostatic cancer that runs in families. If two or more closely related members of your family have had prostatic cancer, especially when they were fairly young, it is probably worth having your prostate checked from time to time once you get to 45 or 50.

I have heard that there is a herbal treatment I can buy at the chemist – wouldn't this be better than having an operation or taking drugs?

There are very many herbal and plant treatments said to help prostate disease. Although not used very much in the UK, they are very popular in some European countries. In fact, the Worldwide Fund for Nature is worried because a species of tree has almost been wiped out because its bark is thought to be an effective treatment for BPH.

Most of these treatments have not been properly tested. If they work it may just be a 'placebo effect' (see page 109).

There is no reason why plants should not make substances that work a bit like the drugs prescribed for BPH. However, these plant substances could have just as many side effects, if not more, than the properly prescribed drugs, so may not be any 'safer'.

If you want to try tablets to help your prostate you should ask your doctor about one of the drugs described on pages 50–2 for BPH. They have been proved to work and to be safe. Also see page 54.

I'm just 50. If I'm so likely to get prostate trouble could I have an operation now to prevent it?

No! A transurethral resection of the prostate (TURP) removes only part of the prostate, so you could still develop BPH or cancer some years later. Complications such as a urethral stricture might occur and be even more of a nuisance. Also, you would likely have retrograde ejaculation for the rest of your life.

I've been referred for some prostate tests in a clinic which is run by a nurse. I've heard she might do the rectal examination of my prostate. Surely this is something only a doctor should do?

Specially trained nurses are being employed more and more to do the tests needed to check the prostate. As they specialise, they become very good at it. Almost everything else that is done in a clinic of this type is done by nurses in other areas. To have a doctor available to do the rectal examination is a bit wasteful of resources.

If a nurse does examine the prostate, it will only be after she or he has been very well trained – just as she or he would be before being entrusted with, say, measuring blood pressure. The nurse will do it many times a week, whereas doctors who don't work in urology departments may need to do it only occasionally.

Although you might feel that a female nurse shouldn't be doing this to a male patient, putting suppositories into the back passage is a very traditional nursing job which isn't really that different.

Will a prostate operation make me infertile?

Most men undergo prostate operations at an age when their partners can no longer have children, and thus issues of fertility and the need for contraception do not arise.

Certainly, complete removal of the prostate, as in a radical prostatectomy for cancer, will inevitably cause infertility and thus, after such an operation, contraception would not be necessary.

A TURP or an open prostatectomy done for benign disease will reduce fertility, particularly if retrograde ejaculation occurs. However, infertility is not inevitable and, if for whatever reason you were using contraceptives before your operation, you would need to continue to do so afterwards.

Case histories

Case history 1: prostate cancer

A man of 68 had had a TURP for BPH some years earlier. He developed further symptoms. When he was examined, his prostate was small but was very hard, and some tissue taken from it showed cancer.

It was planned to give radiotherapy to the prostate, but a bone scan showed that there were a few small areas of cancer in the spine. These were causing no symptoms and as he was well and his prostate was no longer giving him trouble, he decided that he would prefer not to be treated.

He knew that it was important to be closely watched and he was seen by the urologist every few months and his PSA measured. Over the next 15 months, his PSA slowly started to rise, and his prostate symptoms came back.

Although his bone scan had not altered, it was decided that he should have some hormone treatment. As he did not fancy losing his potency he was treated with bicalutamide. His prostate symptoms improved and, within three months, the PSA had become completely normal.

All remained well for 18 months, when the PSA started to rise again. He was started on injections of an LHRH drug, and then the bicalutamide was stopped. He remains well and his PSA has fallen a little once more.

Comments and observations
This tells us a lot about cancer of the prostate. As cancer develops in the outer part of the prostate, having a TURP for BPH does not mean that cancer can't develop later.

Where the disease is detected at a fairly early stage, having a delay in treatment may not matter. This reduces the risk of side effects, as also does choosing the right treatment for the patient – bicalutamide because he wanted to remain potent. Although the effect of hormone treatment is not permanent, changing treatment is sometimes helpful.

Although this man has been quite lucky, he has kept well for several years, showing that cancer of the prostate, even when it cannot be cured, can often be kept under control. As treatment is effective, it is important to keep outpatient appointments, especially if treatment has been deferred.

Note the amount of choice this man had about his treatment.

Case history 2: retention of urine
A man of 90 attended a urologist because he was having trouble passing his urine. His prostate felt quite large. His PSA was measured and was almost 40 (10 times the normal level). This is usually considered to mean that there is definitely cancer in the prostate.

As he was so old and not very fit, the best treatment was difficult to decide, but meanwhile he came into hospital with retention of urine and needed a catheter. As he could not pass urine when the catheter was removed, it was decided he should have an operation and, because the prostate was so large, it had to be taken out at an open operation.

The prostate was found to weigh 350 grams. As most enlarged prostates are less than 40–50 grams this was very large indeed. The pathology examination confirmed it to be BPH with no evidence of cancer.

Comments and observations

An open operation (see page 41), although a bit old fashioned, is still the best way to deal with a very large prostate.

In BPH, the level of PSA depends on the size of the gland. If the gland is unusually large, like this man's, the PSA will also be much higher than would be expected for BPH.

This emphasises the problems of using PSA to diagnose cancer.

Case history 3: bladder tumour

A man was admitted for a prostate operation for which he had been waiting for a few months. Two days before admission, for the first time ever, he noticed some blood in his urine.

Although the bleeding had stopped, the urologist did a careful cystoscopy examination of the bladder before starting the actual TURP and found a small tumour in the lining of the bladder, which was simple to remove at the same time.

Comments and observations

It is never safe to assume that bleeding is from the prostate, even if the prostate is causing other symptoms. If another cause is found, it is most often a bladder tumour. Although there is no connection between bladder tumours and BPH, it is very common, so a lot of men with bladder tumours will also have BPH.

Case history 4: urethral stricture

A man of 65 complained of difficulty passing urine about six months after a heart operation (a coronary artery bypass graft performed for angina). His prostate was enlarged and he was referred to a urologist to see if a prostate operation was needed.

The urologist did a cystoscopy and found a stricture in the urethra. This was cut open by a small operation called a urethrotomy, which is done with an instrument similar to that used to do a TURP.

This completely cured his symptoms, even though his prostate was enlarged.

Comments and observations

Other things can cause prostate-type symptoms, so even if the prostate feels enlarged it may not be the cause of trouble. A catheter is used during heart operations to help check that enough urine is coming. The urologist knew that this can occasionally cause a urethral stricture and advised a cystoscopy examination.

Case history 5: submeatal stricture

Two months after a TURP, the patient felt that his symptoms were coming back and noticed that his urine was spraying as it left the tip of his penis. He went back to the urologist who diagnosed a short stricture just behind the external urinary opening.

This was gently stretched with some metal dilators and, after this had been done a few times, the patient has had no more trouble.

Comments and observations
Called a submeatal stricture, this is not unusual after a TURP and is easily treated. Don't despair if all is not going completely smoothly after a prostate operation. Many of the problems are simple to put right.

Case history 6: raised PSA
Having had mild prostate symptoms for a few years, a man of 70 saw his GP because he had suddenly become worse. A blood test was done, and his PSA was 10 – significantly raised although not very high. It suggested the possibility of cancer.

He saw a urologist three weeks later, who examined the prostate, which felt benign, and retested the PSA, which was 7. This was reassuring and, two months later, not only had the PSA returned to normal but the patient's symptoms had also resolved and nothing more needed to be done.

Comments and observations
This man clearly had some sudden event affecting his prostate, perhaps a mild infection, or a little internal bleeding sufficient to cause bruising or swelling without external evidence of blood. Sometimes a large prostate can lose part of its blood supply and the 'dead' area causes temporary swelling. Some urologists believe this is what happens to men who suddenly get retention when they have had no previous trouble.

When something like this happens, PSA is released into the blood and increases the amount measured. Just because a single PSA measurement is high, it is wrong to jump to conclusions about cancer. Indeed, BPH alone could cause the level of PSA found at first in this man.

Case history 7: acute prostatitis

A man of 58 returned from a dinner party. When he passed urine he had severe burning pain and noticed his urine stream was poor. He had a sudden shivering attack. A few hours later his temperature was 39°C.

He called his doctor who started him on antibiotics. He felt better, but continued to have difficulty passing urine. When it almost completely stopped, he saw a urologist who advised immediate admission to hospital. His prostate was hard but also tender. His PSA was 25 (six times normal).

A catheter was passed and the antibiotics continued. After a few days he was able to pass urine when the catheter was removed, but still with some difficulty. He continued to take antibiotics.

His symptoms gradually improved and his PSA fell, although it was two months before it was back to normal. When he had completely recovered, his prostate felt soft and benign once more, but his urine flow rate was still well below normal.

Comments and observations

This man had severe acute prostatitis. Despite not being aware of it, the fact that his flow rate on recovery was reduced probably means that he already had some obstruction from his prostate and the swelling from the prostatitis pushed him into retention.

Acute prostatitis can make the prostate feel hard and can cause very high levels of PSA – indeed it may be best not to measure it in this situation. The raised PSA takes a long time to recover.

He took antibiotics for six weeks – stopping the treatment for prostatitis too soon can lead to relapse. It does seem that prostatitis is sometimes precipitated by drinking alcohol.

Useful addresses

Where can I find out more?

We have included the following organisations because, on preliminary investigation, they may be of use to the reader. However, we do not have first-hand experience of each organisation and so cannot guarantee the organisation's integrity. The reader must therefore exercise his or her own discretion and judgement when making further enquiries.

Often the associations listed in this section will have a website. Within the website there may well be a section called 'Links'. Here you will find the addresses of other internet resources that you might find useful

Benefits Enquiry Line
Helpline: 0800 882200 (8.30am–6.30pm)
Minicom: 0800 243355
Website: www.dwp.gov.uk
N. Ireland: 0800 220 674
Minicom: 0800 243787

Government agency giving information and advice on sickness and disability benefits for people with disabilities and their carers.

Cancerbackup (British Association of Cancer United Patients)
3 Bath Place, Rivington Street
London EC2A 3JR
Tel: 020 7696 9003
Fax: 020 7696 9002
Freephone: 0808 800 1234
Helpline: 020 7739 2280
Email: info@cancerbackup.org
Website: www.cancerbackup.org.uk

Offers an information service in several languages staffed by specially trained nurses and supported by a panel of medical specialists, about all aspects of different cancers, treatment and related issues. Gives advice and support to patients and families.

Citizens Advice Bureaux
Myddelton House, 115–123 Pentonville Road
London N1 9LZ
Tel: 020 7833 2181 (admin only)
Website: www.adviceguide.org.uk

HQ of national charity offering a wide variety of
practical, financial and legal advice. Network of local
charities throughout the UK listed in phone books and
in Yellow Pages under 'C'.

Continence Foundation
307 Hatton Square, 16 Baldwins Gardens
London EC1N 7RJ
Tel: 020 7404 6875
Helpline: 0845 345 0165 (Mon–Fri 9.30am–1pm)
Fax: 020 7404 6876
Email: continence-help@dial.pipex.com
Website: www.continence-foundation.org.uk

Offers information to people with bladder and/or
bowel problems. Has list of regional specialists. An SAE
requested. Helpline staffed by specialist nurses.

Macmillan Cancer Support
89 Albert Embankment
London SE1 7UQ
Tel: 020 8563 9800
Fax: 020 8563 9640
Email: cancerline@macmillan.org.uk
Website: www.macmillan.org.uk
Helpline: 0808 808 2020
Textphone: 0808 808 0121

Provides information and support for people with cancer and their families. Funds NHS Macmillan nurses for home care as well as hospital and hospice support. Financial help may also be given. Local support groups.

NHS Direct
Tel: 0845 4647 (24 hours, 365 days a year)
Textphone: 0845 606 4647
Website: www.nhsdirect.nhs.uk
NHS Scotland: 0800 224488

Offers confidential health-care advice, information and referral service. A good first port of call for any health advice.

NHS Smoking Helpline
Tel: 0800 169 0169 (7am–11pm, 365 days a year)
Pregnancy smoking helpline: 0800 169 9169
(12 noon–9pm, 365 days a year)
Website: www.givingupsmoking.co.uk

Have advice, help and encouragement on giving up smoking. Specialist advisers available to offer on-going support to those who genuinely are trying to give up smoking. Can refer to local branches.

National Institute for Health and Clinical Excellence (NICE)
MidCity Place, 71 High Holborn
London WC1V 6NA
Tel: 020 7067 5800
Fax: 020 7067 5801
Email: nice@nice.nhs.uk
Website: www.nice.org.uk

Provides national guidance on the promotion of good health and the prevention and treatment of ill-health. Patient information leaflets are available for each piece of guidance issued.

Prodigy Website
Sowerby Centre for Health Informatics at Newcastle (SCHIN), Bede House, All Saints Business Centre
Newcastle upon Tyne NE1 2ES
Tel: 0191 243 6100
Fax: 0191 243 6101
Email: prodigy-enquiries@schin.co.uk
Website: www.prodigy.nhs.uk

A website mainly for GPs giving information for patients listed by disease plus named self-help organisations.

Prostate Cancer Charity
3 Angel Walk, Hammersmith
London W6 9HX
Tel: 020 8222 7622
Fax: 020 8222 7639
Helpline: 0800 074 8383 (Mon–Fri 10am–4pm and Wed eve 7–9 pm)
Textphone: 0845 300 8484
Email: info@prostate-cancer.org.uk
Website: www.prostate-cancer.org.uk

Experienced nurses offer confidential advice and information via helpline, email and face to face. Can refer to network of individuals locally who have had personal experience of the disorder.

Prostate Cancer Research Centre
3rd Floor, 67 Riding House Street
London W1W 7EJ
Tel/fax: 020 7679 9366
Email: info@prostate-cancer-research.org.uk
Website: www.ucl.ac.uk/prostate-cancer-research.org.uk

Publishes a free booklet *The Treatment of Prostate Cancer: Questions and answers*. Raises money for research into prostate cancer.

Prostate Cancer Support Association
BM Box 9434
London WC1N 3XX
Helpline: 0845 601 0766
Email: helpline@prostatecancersupport.information
Website: www.prostatecancersupport.co.uk

Association of self-help and support groups managed by and for men with prostate cancer and their families. Volunteers offer information on treatments and support to anybody affected by cancer. Can refer to local groups in your area.

Prostate Research Campaign UK
10 Northfields Prospect, Putney Bridge Road
London SW18 1PE
Tel: 020 8877 5840
Fax: 020 8877 2609
Email: info@prostate-research.org.uk
Website: www.prostate-research.org.uk

Offers information, free fact sheets and leaflets, about all prostate diseases. Videos and DVDs for sale.

Quit (Smoking Quitlines)
211 Old Street
London EC1V 9NR
Tel: 020 7251 1551
Fax: 020 7251 1661
Helpline: 0800 002200 (9am–9pm, 365 days a year)
Email: info@quit.org.uk
Website: www.quit.org.uk
Scotland: 0800 848484
Wales: 0800 169 0169 (NHS)

Offers individual advice on giving up smoking in
English and Asian languages. Talks to schools on
smoking and pregnancy and can refer to local support
groups. Runs training courses for professionals.

**Scottish Association of Prostate Cancer Support
Groups (SPCa)**
Algo Business Centre, Glenearn Road
Perth PH2 0NJ
Tel/fax: 01738 450415 (Mon–Wed, Fri
9.30am–12.30pm)
Email: supportprostate@tiscali.co.uk
Website: www.prostatescot.co.uk

Has a network of nine Scottish regional groups
providing information, literature and practical support
to men affected by prostate cancer and their families.

Sexual Dysfunction Association
Windmill Place Business Centre, 2–4 Windmill Lane
Southall, Middx UB2 4NJ
Helpline: 0870 774 3571

Email: info@sda.uk.net
Website: www.sda.uk.net

Runs an information helpline, publishes leaflets and offers advice on referral services for all sexual dysfunction problems.

Websites
www.bbc.co.uk/health/conditions/prostatecancer/ shtml
BBC Health

www.bps-assoc.org.uk
British Prostatitis Support Association
Internet-based information and support offered by volunteers to other sufferers of prostate-related disease.

www.chronicprostatitis.com
Independent, volunteer-run site offering cutting-edge information.

The internet as a source of further information
After reading this book, you may feel that you would like further information on the subject. The internet is of course an excellent place to look and there are many websites with useful information about medical disorders, related charities and support groups.

For those who do not have a computer at home some bars and cafes offer facilities for accessing the internet. These are listed in the *Yellow Pages* under 'Internet Bars and Cafes' and 'Internet Providers'. Your local library offers a similar facility and has staff to help you find the information that you need.

It should always be remembered, however, that the internet is unregulated and anyone is free to set up a website and add information to it. Many websites offer impartial advice and information that has been compiled and checked by qualified medical professionals. Some, on the other hand, are run by commercial organisations with the purpose of promoting their own products. Others still are run by pressure groups, some of which will provide carefully assessed and accurate information whereas others may be suggesting medications or treatments that are not supported by the medical and scientific community.

Unless you know the address of the website you want to visit – for example, www.familydoctor.co.uk – you may find the following guidelines useful when searching the internet for information.

Search engines and other searchable sites

Google (www.google.co.uk) is the most popular search engine used in the UK, followed by Yahoo! (http://uk.yahoo.com) and MSN (www.msn.co.uk). Also popular are the search engines provided by Internet Service Providers such as Tiscali and other sites such as the BBC site (www.bbc.co.uk).

In addition to the search engines that index the whole web, there are also medical sites with search facilities, which act almost like mini-search engines, but cover only medical topics or even a particular area of medicine. Again, it is wise to look at who is responsible for compiling the information offered to ensure that it is impartial and medically accurate. The NHS Direct site (www.nhsdirect.nhs.uk) is an example of a searchable medical site.

Links to many British medical charities can be found at the Association of Medical Research Charities' website (www.amrc.org.uk) and at Charity Choice (www.charitychoice.co.uk).

Search phrases

Be specific when entering a search phrase. Searching for information on 'cancer' will return results for many different types of cancer as well as on cancer in general. You may even find sites offering astrological information. More useful results will be returned by using search phrases such as 'lung cancer' and 'treatments for lung cancer'. Both Google and Yahoo! offer an advanced search option that includes the ability to search for the exact phrase; enclosing the search phrase in quotes, that is, 'treatments for lung cancer', will have the same effect. Limiting a search to an exact phrase reduces the number of results returned but it is best to refine a search to an exact match only if you are not getting useful results with a normal search. Adding 'UK' to your search term will bring up mainly British sites, so a good phrase might be 'lung cancer' UK (don't include UK within the quotes).

Always remember the internet is international and unregulated. It holds a wealth of valuable information but individual sites may be biased, out of date or just plain wrong. Family Doctor Publications accepts no responsibility for the content of links published in this series.

Index

abscesses 103

active surveillance 78, 85, 121

acute prostatitis 102–3
 – case history 126–7
 – *see also* prostatitis

acute retention of urine 12–13, 56–7

advanced prostate cancer 88
 – bisphosphonates 97–8
 – case history 121–2
 – chemotherapy 97
 – hormone treatments 88–96
 – radiotherapy 96–7

age, relationship to prostate problems 114

ageing, effects on organs 22

alcohol consumption 127

alfuzosin (Xatral) 50

alpha-blocker drugs 49–50, 55, 57
 – use in combined treatment 51

 – use in prostatodynia 104

ambulatory urodynamics 36

anaesthetics
 – for catheterisation 56, 57
 – for TURP 44

anaemia 88

androgens 90
 – *see also* testosterone

anti-androgens 94–5

anti-inflammatory drugs 104

antibiotics 103, 105, 106, 126, 127

artificial sphincters 80

Association of Medical Research Charities 137

asymptomatic infections 105–6

attitudes to prostate problems 1–2

availability of new treatments 53–4

Avodart (dutasteride) 48, 49, 51, 107

Benefits Enquiry Line 129
benign prostatic hyperplasia
        (BPH) 3, 14–15, 16
– case history 122–3
– difference from prostate
    cancer 68
– occurrence in older men
    114
– open access clinics
    111–12
– prevention 107, 116
– treatment 40–1, 55
    – drugs 48–52
    – heat treatment 52
    – herbal remedies 54, 118
    – laser treatment 52–3
    – stents 54
    – transurethral resection
        of the prostate 41–8
– treatment by GPs 110–11
– variability of symptoms
    114–15
bicalutamide (Casodex) 95,
    121, 122
biopsies 34, 61–2, 69
bisphosphonates 97–8
bladder
– control of urine flow 9
– effect of prostate
    enlargement 11
– effect of radiotherapy 82
bladder stones 14, 21
bladder tumours 21, 23
– case history 123–4
bleeding 14, 21, 23, 24
– case history 123–4
– investigation 32, 36
– after investigations 38, 39
– during radical
    prostatectomy 80

– after radiotherapy 82
– after TURP 44–5, 45–6
– value of hormone
    treatments 49
blood in semen 115
blood tests 30
– in clinical trials 109
– *see also* prostate-specific
    antigen (PSA)
blood transfusions 80
bone pain
– bisphosphonates 97–8
– radiotherapy 96–7
bone scans 71, 121
bones
– effects of hormone
    treatment 93
– spread of prostate cancer
    68, 121
– symptoms of advanced
    cancer 88
bowel, effects of radiotherapy
    82
BPH *see* benign prostatic
    hyperplasia
brachytherapy 76–8, 82–4
British Association of
    Cancer United Patients
    (Cancerbackup) 129
British Prostatitis Support
    Association 135
Brufen (ibuprofen) 104
burning on passing urine 14,
    17, 38, 82, 102, 126
– after radiotherapy 82

cancer *see* prostate cancer
Cancerbackup 129
capsule of prostate 15
Cardura (doxazosin) 50

case histories
- acute prostatitis **126–7**
- bladder tumour **123–4**
- prostate cancer **121–2**
- raised PSA **125–6**
- retention of urine **122–3**
- submeatal stricture **124–5**
- urethral stricture **124**

Casodex (bicalutamide) **95, 121, 122**

catheterisation **56–7, 58**
- during brachytherapy **84**
- as cause of strictures **21, 124**
- during cystometrogram tests **35**
- after radical prostatectomy **80**
- after TURP **44–5**

Charity Choice **137**

check-ups **25**

chemotherapy **97**

chronic pelvic pain syndrome **103–5**

chronic retention of urine **13–14, 57–8**

ciprofloxacin (Ciproxin) **103**

circumcision **29**

Citizens Advice Bureaux **130**

clinical trials **86–7, 108–10**

cold weather **13**

combined drug treatment for BPH **51**

complications of treatment *see* side effects of treatment

conformal radiotherapy **76, 77, 82**

constipation **13**

Continence Foundation **130**

cryotherapy **85**

CT (computed tomography) scans **34**

cyproterone acetate (Cyprostat) **95**

cystitis **102**
- after radiotherapy **82**

cystometrogram test **35–6, 38**

cystoscopy **36–8, 123**

day-case surgery for BPH **53**

Decapeptyl SR (triptorelin) **91**

diabetes **22**

diarrhoea after radiotherapy **82**

diet and prostate cancer **68, 99, 116**

diethylstilbestrol **95**

diuretics **13**

docetaxel **97**

Doralese (indoramin) **50**

double-blind clinical trials **108–9**

doxazosin (Cardura) **50**

dribbling **10**
- after TURP **46**
- *see also* incontinence

driving after TURP **45**

Drogenil (flutamide) **95**

drug treatments for BPH **55**
- alpha-blocker drugs **49–50**
- choice of drug **50–1**
- combined treatment **51**
- hormones **48–9**
- when they are used **51–2**

dutasteride (Avodart) **48, 49, 51, 107**

dysuria **14, 17, 38, 126**
– after radiotherapy **82**

ejaculation, retrograde **46–7, 50, 118**

embarrassment **1, 4**

enlargement of prostate **8, 11**
– causes
– benign prostatic hyperplasia **14–15, 16**
– cancer of prostate **15–16, 17**
– prostatitis **16–17**
– symptoms
– acute retention of urine **12–13**
– chronic retention of urine **13–14**
– storage (irritative) symptoms **10–12**
– voiding (obstructive) symptoms **8, 10**

epididymitis **102, 117**

epithelium/epithelial cells **5, 6, 7, 8**

erection problems
– during hormone treatment **49, 92–3**
– after radical prostatectomy **81**
– after radiotherapy **82**
– after TURP **47**

ethical committees **109**

examination **28–30, 119**

external beam radiotherapy **75–6, 81–2**

external bladder sphincter **9**
– and TURP **43, 47**

family history of prostate cancer **68, 117**

fatty foods **68, 99, 116**

female hormones **95**

fertility, effect of surgery **119–20**

finasteride (Proscar) **48, 49, 51, 99–100, 107**

Flomaxtra XL (tamsulosin) **50**

flow tests **30–2**
– before brachytherapy **84**

fluid intake
– in BPH **116**
– in prostatitis **103**
– after TURP **45**

flutamide (Drogenil) **95**

foreskin, narrowing **28–9**

fractions, radiotherapy **81**

frequency of passing urine **11, 12**
– after TURP **45**

gene therapy **98–9**

geographical differences, prostate cancer **68**

glands **5, 7, 8**

Gleason score **69, 78**

goserelin (Zoladex) **91**

GP
– as source of help **25**
– treatment of prostate problems **110–11**

green light laser treatment **53**

haematuria (blood in urine) **14, 21, 23, 24**
– case history **123–4**
– investigation **32, 36**
– after investigations **38, 39**

haematuria (contd)
- after TURP 44–5, 45–6
- value of hormone treatments 49
heat treatment for BPH 52
help, where to find it 25–6
- searching the internet 135–7
- useful addresses 128–35
- websites 135
herbal remedies for BPH 54, 118
hesitancy 8, 10
hormone treatments
- for BPH 48–9, 50–1, 55
- for cancer of prostate 77, 87–8, 101
- advanced cancer 88–96, 121–2
hormones, effect on prostate 5
hot flushes 93
hyperthermia treatment for BPH 52
Hypovase (prazosin) 50
Hytrin (terazosin) 50

ibuprofen 104
illness, retention of urine 13
immunotherapy 99
impotence see erection problems
incomplete emptying 10, 12
incontinence 11, 12, 14
- Continence Foundation 130
- after radical prostatectomy 80
- after radiotherapy 82
- after TURP 46, 47

indometacin (Indocid) 104
indoramin (Doralese) 50
infections 14
- asymptomatic 105–6
- after biopsy of the prostate 61–2
- prostatitis 16–17, 102–3
- of testicles 117
injections, hormone treatment 91, 94
inner part of prostate 7, 8
- benign prostatic hyperplasia 15, 16
intensity-modulated radiotherapy (IMRT) 76
internal bladder sphincter 9, 43
intravenous urogram (IVU) 23, 32
investigations 30, 39
- cystometrogram 35–6
- cystoscopy 36–8, 123
- magnetic resonance imaging 34–5, 71, 72
- transrectal ultrasound scan 33–4, 61, 69, 70
- before TURP 44
- urine flow measurement 30–2
- X-rays and ultrasound scans 32–3
irritative (storage) symptoms 10–12

keyhole (laparoscopic) surgery 74–5
kidney tumours 23
kidneys
- effect of chronic retention 14, 57–8

– X-rays and ultrasound scans 32

laparoscopic radical prostatectomy 74–5
laser treatment for BPH 52–3
leaking 11, 12, 14
– after radical prostatectomy 80
– after radiotherapy 82
– after TURP 46, 47
leuprorelin (Prostap SR) 91
lifestyle changes 22
lumps in testicles 117
luteinising hormone-releasing hormone (LHRH) analogues 91, 94, 122
lymph nodes, removal 79

Macmillan Cancer Support 130–1
medical advice, when to seek it 25, 26
metastases 16, 68
– see also bone pain
Metastron (strontium-89) therapy 96–7
MRI (magnetic resonance imaging) 34–5, 72
– in prostate cancer 71
muscle fibres 6
– as cause of symptoms 15
– effect of alpha-blocker drugs 49
– spasm 104

National Institute for Health and Clinical Excellence (NICE) 131–2

'natural' remedies for BPH 54
needle biopsies 34, 61–2, 69
new treatments for BPH 52–3
– availability 53–4
NHS Direct 131
NHS Smoking Helpline 131
night time symptoms (nocturia) 11, 12, 22
– persistence after TURP 46
norfloxacin (Utinor) 103
Nurofen (ibuprofen) 104
nurses, specialised 111, 119

obstructive (voiding) symptoms 8, 10
– bladder stones 21
– urethral stricture 19–21
oestrogens 95
ofloxacin (Tarivid) 103
open access clinics 111–12
open surgery 41, 123
operations see surgery
orchiectomy 91, 92, 94
osteoporosis 98
outer part of prostate 7, 8
– cancer 15–16, 17
– effect of benign prostatic hyperplasia 15, 16
overfull bladder 13

pacemakers 34
pain
– chronic pelvic pain syndrome 103–5
– in testicles 117
– after TURP 45
– see also bone pain
pamidronate 98
Parkinson's disease 22

pathological examination, prostate cancer **69**

phimosis **28–9**

physical examination **28–30**

phytoestrogens **99**

piles **29**

pis en deux **10**

pituitary gland **89, 90**

placebos **109, 118**

poor stream **10, 35**

prazosin (Hypovase) **50**

pre-admission clinics **44**

pressure measurements (cystometrogram) **35–6, 38**

prevention of BPH **116, 118**

prevention of prostate cancer **99–100, 116**

Prodigy Website **132**

Proscar (finasteride) **48, 49, 51, 99–100, 107**

Prostap SR (leuprorelin) **91**

prostate
  – anatomy **5–8**
  – what it is **5**

prostate assessment clinics **26–7**
  – describing your symptoms **27–8**
  – examination **28–30**
  – open access clinics **111–12**
  – symptom questionnaires **28**
  – tests **30–8**

prostate cancer **15–16, 17, 65–6, 67**
  – case history **121–2**
  – checking for spread of tumour **71**
  – diagnosis **69**
  – family history of **68, 117**
  – occurrence in older men **114**
  – prevention **99–100, 116, 118**
  – tests **2, 34**
    – PSA **61, 62, 63–4**
  – treatments **71, 108**
    – active surveillance **78**
    – bisphosphonates **97–8**
    – chemotherapy **97**
    – choice of method **79, 85–6, 87**
    – clinical trials **86–7**
    – cryotherapy **85**
    – hormone treatment **87–8, 88–96**
    – laparoscopic radical prostatectomy **74–5**
    – new treatments **98–9**
    – radical prostatectomy **72–4, 79–81**
    – radiotherapy **75–8, 81–4, 96–7**
  – what triggers it **68**

Prostate Cancer Charity **132**

Prostate Cancer Research Centre **133**

Prostate Cancer Support Association **133**

Prostate Research Campaign UK **133–4**

prostate-specific antigen (PSA) **30, 60**
  – in asymptomatic infections **105–6**
  – in prostate cancer **62–3, 69, 79, 121–2**
  – in prostatitis **126–7**

– screening for prostate cancer 63–4

– testing on request 64–5

– when it is high 61, 122–3, 125–6

prostatitis 14, 16–17, 102–3, 115, 116–17

– case history 126–7

– diagnosis 104

– websites 135

prostatodynia 104

PSA *see* prostate-specific antigen

quinolone antibiotics 103

Quit (Smoking Quitlines) 134

racial differences, prostate cancer 68

radical prostatectomy 63, 65–6, 72–4, 101

– complications 80–1

– effect on fertility 119

– laparoscopic 74–5

– what it involves 79–80

radioactive bone scans 71

radiotherapy 101

– for bone pain 96–7

– brachytherapy 76–8

– external beam treatment 75–6, 81–2

randomised clinical trials 86, 108–9

rectal examination 29–30, 119

resectoscopes 42, 43

retention of urine

– acute 12–13, 56–7

– case history 122–3

– chronic 13–14, 57–8

– in prostatitis 102, 126

retirement from work 22

retrograde ejaculation 46–7, 50, 118

robotic prostatectomy 75

Scottish Association of Prostate Cancer Support Groups (SPCa) 134

screening for prostate cancer 2, 63–4

secondary tumour (metastases) 16, 68

– *see also* bone pain

seeds, radioactive 77–8, 82–4

self-assessment questions 26

semen 5, 6

– blood in 115

seminal fluid 6, 7

seminal vesicles 6, 9

Sexual Dysfunction Association 135

sexual intercourse

– after prostatitis 103

– after TURP 45, 46–7

sexual partners 115

sexual problems

– during hormone treatment 49, 92–3

– after radical prostatectomy 81

– after radiotherapy 82

side effects of treatment

– of alpha-blocker drugs 50

– of brachytherapy 78

– of external beam radiotherapy 76–7, 82

– of hormone treatment 49, 92–4, 95

– of radical prostatectomy 80–1

sleep disturbance **11, 22**
smoking
  – NHS Smoking Helpline
    131
  – Quit (Smoking Quitlines)
    134
soya products **68, 99, 116**
specialised nurses **111, 119**
sphincters **9**
  – artificial **80**
  – effect of TURP **43, 47**
spinal anaesthetic **44**
spine, spread of prostate
    cancer **71, 121**
stents **54**
stones in bladder **14, 21**
storage (irritative) symptoms
    10–12, 21–2
strictures **19–21**
  – case histories **124–5**
strokes **22**
stroma **5–6, 7, 8, 15**
strontium-89 (Metastron)
    therapy **96–7**
subcapsular orchiectomy **91,
    92, 94**
submeatal stricture **124–5**
suprapubic catheters **57**
surgery **40–1, 50, 55**
  – for abscesses **103**
  – effect on fertility
    119–20
  – laparoscopic radical
    prostatectomy **74–5**
  – laser treatment **52–3**
  – open operations for BPH
    41, 123
  – preventive **118**
  – radical prostatectomy **63,
    65–6, 72–4, 79–81**

  – removal of testicles **91, 92**
  – after retention of urine
    58–9
  – transurethral resection of
    the prostate (TURP) **41–8**
  – urethrotomy **124**
sweating **93**
symptom questionnaires **28**
symptoms
  – acute retention of urine
    12–13
  – of advanced cancer **88**
  – chronic retention of urine
    13–14
  – describing them to your
    doctor **27–8**
  – storage (irritative)
    symptoms **10–12**
  – variability **114–15**
  – voiding (obstructive)
    symptoms **8, 10**

tamsulosin (Flomaxtra XL) **50**
Tarivid (ofloxacin) **103**
terazosin (Hytrin) **50**
terminal dribbling **10**
  – after TURP **46**
testes (testicles) **6**
  – effects of hormone
    treatment **93**
  – infection of **102**
  – lumps in **117**
  – pain **117**
  – removal of **91**
testosterone **48, 89, 90**
tests **2, 30**
  – cystometrogram **35–6**
  – cystoscopy **36–8, 123**
  – magnetic resonance
    imaging **34–5, 71, 72**

– transrectal ultrasound scan 33–4, 61, 69, 70
– before TURP 44
– urine flow measurement 30–2
– X-rays and ultrasound scans 32–3
thermotherapy for BPH 52
tiredness during hormone treatment 93
tissue in urine 45
transrectal ultrasound scan (TRUS) 33–4, 61, 69, 70
– use in brachytherapy 78, 83, 84
transurethral resection of the prostate (TURP) 41–3, 118, 121, 122
– after the operation 44–8
– effect on fertility 119–20
– examination of removed tissue 69
– having the operation 44
– submeatal strictures 124–5
treatments 3
– for BPH 40–1, 55
– drug treatments 48–52
– heat treatments 52
– herbal remedies 54
– laser treatments 52–3
– stents 54
– transurethral resection of prostate 41–8
– for cancer of prostate 71
– active surveillance 78
– bisphosphonates 97–8
– chemotherapy 97
– choice of method 79, 85–6, 87
– clinical trials 86–7
– cryotherapy 85
– hormone treatment 87–8, 88–96
– laparoscopic radical prostatectomy 74–5
– new treatments 98–9
– radical prostatectomy 72–4, 79–81
– radiotherapy 75–8, 81–4, 96–7
– clinical trials 108–10
– improvements 107
– who will treat you 110
triptorelin (Decapeptyl SR) 91
tumours in bladder 21, 23

ultrasound scans 23, 32, 33
– transrectal ultrasound 33–4, 61, 69, 70
unstable bladder 35
ureters 6
urethra 6, 7
– effect of prostate enlargement 8, 11, 16
urethral stricture 19–21, 38
– case history 124
urethrotomy 124
urgency of passing urine 11, 12
urine
– control of flow from bladder 9
– inability to pass it see retention of urine
urine control
– after radical prostatectomy 80
– after TURP 45, 47

urine flow measurement 30–2
urine infections 14
urine samples 30
urodynamics (cystometrogram) 35–6, 38
urologists 25
urology department referral 26–7
 – describing your symptoms 27–8
 – examination 28–30, 119
 – open access clinics 111–12
 – symptom questionnaires 28
 – tests 30–8
Utinor (norfloxacin) 103

vaporisation treatment 53
vas deferens 6, 9
vasectomy 68, 117
voiding (obstructive) symptoms 8, 10
 – bladder stones 21
 – urethral stricture 19–21

watchful waiting (active surveillance) 78–9, 85, 86, 121
websites 135, 137
 – Prodigy Website 132
weight gain, during hormone treatment 93
weight loss 88
wetting (incontinence) 11, 12, 14
 – after radical prostatectomy 80
 – after radiotherapy 82
 – after TURP 46, 47

X-rays 32
 – CT scans 34
 – intravenous urogram 23
 – in prostate cancer 71
Xatral (alfuzosin) 50

Zoladex (goserelin) 91
zoledronate 98

Your pages

We have included the following pages because they may help you manage your illness or condition and its treatment.

Before an appointment with a health professional, it can be useful to write down a short list of questions of things that you do not understand, so that you can make sure that you do not forget anything.

Some of the sections may not be relevant to your circumstances.

We are always pleased to receive constructive criticism or suggestions about how to improve the books. You can contact us at:

Email: familydoctor@btinternet.com
Letter: Family Doctor Publications
         PO Box 4664
         Poole
         BH15 1NN

Thank you

Health-care contact details

Name:

Job title:

Place of work:

Tel:

Name:

Job title:

Place of work:

Tel:

Name:

Job title:

Place of work:

Tel:

Name:

Job title:

Place of work:

Tel:

Significant past health events – illnesses/operations/investigations/treatments

Event	Month	Year	Age (at time)

Appointments for health care

Name:

Place:

Date:

Time:

Tel:

Name:

Place:

Date:

Time:

Tel:

Name:

Place:

Date:

Time:

Tel:

Name:

Place:

Date:

Time:

Tel:

Appointments for health care

Name:

Place:

Date:

Time:

Tel:

Name:

Place:

Date:

Time:

Tel:

Name:

Place:

Date:

Time:

Tel:

Name:

Place:

Date:

Time:

Tel:

Current medication(s) prescribed by your doctor

Medicine name:

Purpose:

Frequency & dose:

Start date:

End date:

Medicine name:

Purpose:

Frequency & dose:

Start date:

End date:

Medicine name:

Purpose:

Frequency & dose:

Start date:

End date:

Medicine name:

Purpose:

Frequency & dose:

Start date:

End date:

Other medicines/supplements you are taking, not prescribed by your doctor

Medicine/treatment:

Purpose:

Frequency & dose:

Start date:

End date:

Medicine/treatment:

Purpose:

Frequency & dose:

Start date:

End date:

Medicine/treatment:

Purpose:

Frequency & dose:

Start date:

End date:

Medicine/treatment:

Purpose:

Frequency & dose:

Start date:

End date:

Questions to ask at appointments
(Note: do bear in mind that doctors work under great time pressure, so long lists may not be helpful for either of you)

Questions to ask at appointments
(Note: do bear in mind that doctors work under great time pressure, so long lists may not be helpful for either of you)

Notes

Notes

Notes